# Women's Health and Complementary and Integrative Medicine

Complementary and integrative medicine (CIM) has become big business internationally, in particular with regards to a range of women's health issues. With this context in mind, *Women's Health and Complementary and Integrative Medicine* constitutes a valuable and timely resource for those looking to understand, initiate and expand CIM research and evidence-based debate with regards to a wide range of women's health care issues.

The collection brings together leading international CIM researchers from Australia, the USA, the UK, Germany and Canada, with backgrounds and expertise in health social science, biostatistics, qualitative methodology, clinical trial design, clinical pharmacology, health services research and public health. Contributors draw upon their own CIM research work and experience to explain and review core research and practice issues pertinent to the contemporary field of CIM and its future development with regards to women's health.

The book outlines the core issues, challenges and opportunities facing the CIM-women's health field and its study and provides insight and inspiration for those practising, studying and/or researching the contemporary relations between CIM and women's health and health care.

**Jon Adams** is Distinguished Professor of Public Health, ARC Professorial Fellow and Director, Australian Research Centre in Complementary and Integrative Medicine (ARCCIM), University of Technology Sydney, Australia.

**Amie Steel** is Postdoctoral Research Fellow, Australian Research Centre in Complementary and Integrative Medicine (ARCCIM), University of Technology Sydney, Australia, and Associate Director of Research, Endeavour College of Natural Health, Australia.

**Alex Broom** is Professor of Sociology, University of New South Wales, Australia, and a Visiting Professor, Australian Research Centre in Complementary and Integrative Medicine (ARCCIM), University of Technology Sydney, Australia.

**Jane Frawley** is an NHMRC Early Career Fellow and Research Fellow, Australian Research Centre in Complementary and Integrative Medicine (ARCCIM), University of Technology Sydney, Australia.

**Routledge Studies in Public Health**
https://www.routledge.com/Routledge-Studies-in-Public-Health/book-series/RSPH

Available titles include:

**Assembling Health Rights in Global Context**
Geneologies and Anthropologies
*Edited by Alex Mould and David Reubi*

**Empowerment, Health Promotion and Young People**
A Critical Approach
*Grace Spencer*

**Risk Communication and Infectious Diseases in an Age of Digital Media**
*Edited by Anat Gesser-Edelsburg and Yaffa Shir-Raz*

**Youth Drinking Cultures in a Digital World**
Alcohol, Social Media and Cultures of Intoxication
*Edited by Antonia Lyons, Tim McCreanor, Ian Goodwin and Helen Moewaka Barnes*

**Global Health Geographies**
*Edited by Clare Herrick and David Reubi*

**The Intersection of Food and Public Health**
Current Policy Challenges and Solutions
*Edited by A. Bryce Hoflund, John C. Jones and Michelle Pautz*

**Conceptualising Public Health**
Historical and Contemporary Struggles over Key Concepts
*Edited by Johannes Kananen, Sophy Bergenheim and Merle Wessel*

**Global Health and Security**
Critical Feminist Perspectives
*Edited by Colleen O'Manique and Pieter Fourie*

**Women's Health and Complementary and Integrative Medicine**
*Edited by Jon Adams, Amie Steel, Alex Broom and Jane Frawley*

# Women's Health and Complementary and Integrative Medicine

Edited by
Jon Adams, Amie Steel, Alex
Broom and Jane Frawley

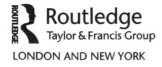
Routledge
Taylor & Francis Group

LONDON AND NEW YORK

First published 2019 by Routledge

2 Park Square, Milton Park, Abingdon, Oxfordshire OX14 4RN

52 Vanderbilt Avenue, New York, NY 10017

*Routledge is an imprint of the Taylor & Francis Group, an informa business*

First issued in paperback 2019

*British Library Cataloguing-in-Publication Data*
A catalogue record for this book is available from the British Library

*Library of Congress Cataloging-in-Publication Data*
Names: Adams, Jon, 1971– editor. | Steel, Amie editor. | Broom, Alex, editor. | Frawley, Jane editor.
Title: Women's health and complementary and integrative medicine / edited by Jon Adams, Amie Steel, Alex Broom, and Jane Frawley.
Other titles: Routledge studies in public health.
Description: Abingdon, Oxon ; New York, NY : Routledge, 2019. | Series: Routledge studies in public health | Includes bibliographical references and index.
Identifiers: LCCN 2018003551| ISBN 9781138959262 (hardback) | ISBN 9781315660721 (ebook)
Subjects: | MESH: Women's Health | Complementary Therapies—methods | Integrative Medicine—methods
Classification: LCC RA564.85 | NLM WA 309.1 | DDC 362.1082—dc23
LC record available at https://lccn.loc.gov/2018003551

ISBN: 978-1-138-95926-2 (hbk)
ISBN: 978-0-367-45754-9 (pbk)

Typeset in Times New Roman
by Florence Production Ltd, Stoodleigh, Devon, UK

# Contents

**PART II**
## CIM use and women's health issues 61

**PART III**
## CIM use, women and the health care system 111

# Tables

# Contributors

**Jon Adams** is Distinguished Professor of Public Health and Director of the Australian Research Centre in Complementary and Integrative Medicine (ARCCIM), University of Technology Sydney, Australia. He is also an Australian Research Council (ARC) Professorial Future Fellow and a Senior Fellow on the International Oxford Primary Care Research Leadership Program, University of Oxford, UK. Jon has previously co-edited seven academic research books including holding Chief Editorship of the first reader collection on *Traditional, Complementary and Integrative Medicine* (Palgrave). He has authored over 370 publications to date and his diverse health research interests include examining issues around primary health care, chronic illness and a range of informal and self-care health-seeking behaviours and practices. More recently, he has also been extensively engaged in implementation and translation research, practice-based research network design and developing strategies and programmes in research capacity building and mentorship.

**Abigail Aiyepola** is the Secretary of the Midwifery Education and Accreditation Council and Associate Dean of the School of Naturopathic Medicine, Maryland University of Integrative Health, USA. Her experience within the realm of higher education is unique in its interdisciplinary nature and spans both the naturopathic and midwifery professions.

**Lise Alschuler** is a naturopath with board certification in naturopathic oncology and has been practising since 1994. She has been President, American Association of Naturopathic Physicians and is the current President of the Oncology Association of Naturopathic Physicians, USA. She works as an independent consultant in the area of practitioner and consumer health education and is a sought-after speaker for professional and lay audiences on various subjects within integrative healthcare.

**Gavin J. Andrews** is Professor and Graduate Chair of the Department of Health, Aging and Society, McMaster University, Canada. He is a leading health geographer and his wide-ranging research explores the dynamics between space/place and: aging, holistic medicine, health care work, phobias, sports and fitness, health histories and popular music. Much of his work is positional and considers the progress, state-of-the-art and future of health geography.

**Alex Broom** is Professor of Sociology and Co-Director of the Practical Justice Initiative at the University of New South Wales (UNSW), Sydney, Australia. He is recognised as an international leader in the sociology of health and illness, with a current focus on developing critical analyses of the social dynamics of cancer and palliative care and the global challenge of antimicrobial resistance. Before joining UNSW, he was an ARC Future Fellow at the University of Queensland from 2011–2015.

**Irena Connon** is a social anthropologist and transdisciplinary researcher in the fields of political ecology, socio-cultural dimensions of resilience and adaptation to environmental hazard events, environmental sustainability and water security. She specialises in qualitative, ethnographic, trans-disciplinary research as well as applied-action and mixed method research designs.

**Holger Cramer** is Research Director, Department of Internal and Integrative Medicine, University of Duisburg-Essen, Germany. He also holds a Visiting Fellowship at the Australian Research Centre in Complementary and Integrative Medicine (ARCCIM), University of Technology Sydney and the International Complementary Medicine Research Leadership Program. Holger has authored more than 100 scientific journal articles on complementary and integrative medicine.

**Peter N. DeMaio** is reading for the MSc in Evidence-Based Social Intervention and Policy Evaluation at McMaster University, Canada. Peter holds a Combined Honours degree in Health Studies and Gerontology and a Master of Arts in Health Studies and Gerontology from McMaster University. Peter was awarded the R.C. McIvor Medal as the top undergraduate scholar in the Faculty of Social Sciences' graduating class of 2015. Peter has worked for the McMaster Health Forum where his primary responsibilities involved supporting the Health Systems Evidence (HSE) – the world's most comprehensive, free access point for evidence to support policy-makers, stakeholders and researchers interested in how to strengthen or reform health systems or in how to get cost-effective programs, services and drugs to those who need them.

**Roger Dunston** is Associate Professor in the Faculty of Arts and Social Science and a member of the International Research Centre for Communication in Healthcare (IRCCH), University of Technology Sydney, Australia. Roger's diverse research interests include examination of the nature of professional practice, making change and service redesign, 'patient' participation and co-production, and professional learning. He has led a number of large national development and research projects in these areas.

**Jane Frawley** is a National Health and Medical Research Council (NHMRC) Early Career Fellow. She is a member of the Australian Centre of Public and Population Health Research and the Australian Research Centre in Complementary and Integrative Medicine (ARCCIM), University of Technology Sydney, Australia. Jane's programme of research within public health epidemiology has a particular focus on maternal and child health.

**Helen Hall** is a Senior Lecturer and the Head of Nursing and Midwifery at the Peninsula campus, Monash University, Australia. Helen's research interests revolve around her work in maternity care with a focus on the use of integrative medical approaches. Helen holds a Visiting Research Fellowship at the Australian Research Centre in Complementary and Integrative Medicine (ARCCIM), University of Technology Sydney, Australia. She is particularly committed to education and research that improves the health outcomes of vulnerable populations.

**Joanna Harnett** is Associate Lecturer, Faculty of Pharmacy, University of Sydney, Australia, where she teaches and researches the broader area of complementary medicines with a focus on fostering their appropriate and safe use and building the evidence base. Joanna is a Fellow of the International Naturopathy Research Leadership Program at the Australian Research Centre in Complementary and Integrative Medicine (ARCCIM), University of Technology Sydney, Australia. Her research projects have focused on probiotic use, health literacy and disclosure of complementary medicine use by Australians, pharmacists' role in fostering the safe and appropriate use of complementary medicine, the practice behaviours of complementary medicine health practitioners, and complementary medicine use in specific populations.

**Romy Lauche** is a Chancellor's Post-Doctoral Research Fellow at the Australian Research Centre in Complementary and Integrative Medicine (ARCCIM), University of Technology Sydney, Australia. Romy has a background and qualifications in psychology and received her PhD in medical sciences. She has extensive experience in clinical research and evidence synthesis, with a focus on chronic illnesses, and the impact of mindfulness and traditional medicine interventions on health and well-being. She currently applies her advanced methodological and statistical skills to conduct public health research in the areas of women's health, mental health and chronic illness.

**Matthew Leach** is a Senior Research Fellow, Department of Rural Health, University of South Australia. He is also a Registered Nurse and naturopath. He is focused upon improving the evidence base and quality of complementary medicine and has made an original and significant contribution to the field over the past decade. He has published over 90 journal articles, four book chapters and a sole-authored textbook, and has attracted over 1120 citations for his work. He is also a Visiting Research Fellow of the Australian Research Centre for Complementary and Integrative Medicine (ARCCIM), University of Technology Sydney, Australia and a Fellow on the International Complementary Medicine Research Leadership Program.

**Ellen McDonell** is a naturopath focusing on integrative cancer care. She is also involved with the research department at the Ottawa Integrative Cancer Centre, Canada, where she works to bridge the gap between conventional and alternative healthcare by studying the effects of an integrative approach to cancer care.

**Erica McIntyre** is a Postdoctoral Research Fellow at the Australian Research Centre in Complementary and Integrative Medicine (ARCCIM), University of Technology Sydney, Australia. Erica has a background in Western herbal medicine and is a Fellow of the ARCCIM International Naturopathy Research Leadership Program. She holds a PhD in psychology, with research interests in the areas of mental health and well-being, health services use, complementary self-care, health communication and decision-making.

**Wenbo Peng** is a Postdoctoral Research Associate at the Australian Research Centre in Complementary and Integrative Medicine (ARCCIM), University of Technology Sydney, Australia, and a registered Chinese herbal medicine practitioner, acupuncturist, and Chinese herbal dispenser in Australia. She was awarded the Barbara Gross Award at the 18th Congress of the Australian Menopause Society in 2014. Dr Peng's research focuses upon public health and health services research, practice-based research networks, women's health, and complementary and traditional medicine.

**Jason Prior** is an Associate Professor, Research Director and Associate Director of the Postgraduate Program at the Institute for Sustainable Futures (ISF), University of Technology Sydney, Australia. Jason's programme of research focuses on processes of spatial governance through a range of techniques including law, architecture, property rights, planning, and environmental management. His more recent collaboration in transdisciplinary research teams examines the built environment, well-being, chronic illness and ageing.

**Catherine Rickwood** is the Founder and CEO of the Three Sisters Group, a consultancy and advisory company providing services for organisations for the over-50s market. She is a member of the Australian Association of Gerontology.

**Janet Schloss** is a naturopath and nutritionist who has been in private practice for over 15 years and completed her doctorate at the School of Medicine, University of Queensland, Australia, through the Princess Alexandra Hospital. She has also lectured in naturopathy at the Endeavour College of Natural Health and her main specialty is naturopathy and people who have cancer and chronic diseases, especially those going through traditional treatment.

**David Sibbritt** is Professor of Epidemiology and Deputy Director, Australian Research Centre in Complementary and Integrative Medicine (ARCCIM), University of Technology Sydney, Australia. He is a world-leading critical public health researcher focusing on complementary and integrative health care. David's research focus has been on women's use of complementary and alternative medicine to treat chronic illness and for their general well-being. He has editorial roles for several international peer-reviewed journals.

**Amie Steel** is a naturopath, educator and researcher in the field of complementary medicine. Amie currently holds dual research positions as a Postdoctoral Research Fellow at the Australian Research Centre in Complementary and

Integrative Medicine (ARCCIM), University of Technology Sydney, and also Associate Director, Office of Research, Endeavour College of Natural Health, Australia. Amie also holds an affiliate faculty position at the Helfgott Research Institute, National University of Natural Medicine in Portland, USA.

# Introduction

*Jon Adams, Amie Steel, Alex Broom and Jane Frawley*

The relationship between women's health and complementary and integrative medicine (CIM) has long been identified as both having a significant bearing upon the activities, behaviours and development in this area of health care (Adams et al. 2003b) and as an important sub-topic worthy of enquiry within the wider CIM and health research project (Adams et al. 2003a; Flesch 2007). In fact, in many regards, it can be seen that the origins and rise of CIM and the health and health-seeking needs and practices of women have been closely connected or even inextricably linked. Women are often cited as keen supporters of CIM and are more likely to be users than men (Bishop and Lewith 2010; Steel et al. 2013; Zhang et al. 2015). In addition, there are a number of women's health issues that lend themselves to CIM use (with a fair number such as women's cancers, pregnancy and menopause reflected in the chapters of this collection). Moreover, CIM practice sites and professional projects are themselves, in many cases, a female-dominated terrain and some commentators have highlighted the potential for CIM to foster new models of health care and/or female-orientated approaches to health.

CIM here refers to a vast range of practices, technologies and products that traditionally exist beyond the scope of the medical profession and medical curriculum (Adams et al. 2012) and which in contemporary care remain primarily but to different degrees outside (state-funded) conventional and allied health care systems. Examples of CIM are therapies and practices led by a range of CIM practitioners including acupuncturists, chiropractors, massage therapists, osteopaths, or naturopaths. Alongside such professionally-led treatments and practices one finds also a wide range of CIM self-care activities and products, such as yoga, meditation, herbal medicine and dietary supplements that require only minimal, if any, input and guidance from a health professional, whether versed in conventional medicine, complementary medicine or both. The chapters in this book cover discussion, empirical analyses and critical evaluation with examples from both of these practitioner-led and women-led CIM subfields.

A current web search of international research attests to a more recent explosion of interest and empirical study on women within the growing CIM research field, with work addressing a vast range of specific research questions and health and health care issues. While some of the core research questions posed by earlier scholars (Adams et al. 2003a) do appear to have received attention in more recent years, there has also been rich investigation on a much broader multi-disciplinary front, accommodating designs, thinking and evaluation from across health services research, public health research, clinical research, and beyond. The broadening of disciplinary and methodological interest in women's health and CIM, a trend in line with all health research in recent times, is reflected across the collection of chapters presented here.

## The structure of the book

The aim of *Women's Health and Complementary and Integrative Medicine* is to introduce a multi-disciplinary, eclectic readership to a number of pertinent and timely substantive topics at the intersect of CIM and women's health. The growing interest in this field as a worthy research topic is essentially international in scope, and, in response, the collection brings together contributors from Australia, Canada, Germany, the UK and the USA. Authors have also been purposefully selected for their spread of disciplinary groundings and expertise, including biostatistics, epidemiology and public health research, health services research, health social science and CIM therapy, among others.

It is interesting to note that CIM use and practice are appearing in a number of health sites and with regards to a range of conditions and time periods across women's life cycle. The book is divided into three Parts. Part I, 'CIM use and women's life cycle', begins with Chapter 1, where Steel and colleagues outline CIM use with regards to the research area of preconception care. As these authors attest, the relationship between CIM use and preconception is a potentially fruitful one, providing both clinically relevant and promising interventions as well as additional tools with which to approach what is still a largely uncharted and only recently emerging topic of empirical enquiry more generally.

In contrast, Frawley and colleagues overview the now somewhat relatively well-trodden research path examining CIM use for pregnancy, labour and birth in Chapter 2. Indeed, this topic has attracted two international critical reviews and has been the subject of some of the largest longitudinal cohort projects in CIM use and women's health to date, drawing upon the Australian Longitudinal Study on Women's Health Sub-study (Adams et al. 2015; Steel et al. 2012) and the Avon Longitudinal Study of Parents and Children, in the UK (Bishop et al. 2011). Nevertheless, as with all health and health care topics, the opportunity to ask more revealing questions and conduct further novel enquiry on pregnancy and CIM remains and, as Chapter 9 in this collection highlights, midwives and doulas have often been the most conspicuous supporters of CIM practices (if not always supporters of CIM practitioners) for women in their care.

In Chapter 3, Peng and colleagues examine the empirical evidence for the efficacy of CIM treatments in the menopause as well as the prevalence, patterns and decision-making of menopausal women regarding CIM use. The chapter introduces contemporary guidelines on CIM use and outlines implications of a number of noteworthy clinical and practice-based issues regarding CIM provision in menopausal care.

The numbers of the ageing population and a range of associated health challenges are taxing health care systems across the globe and it is no surprise that CIM use is a fast emerging research topic with regards to older women. Chapter 4 by Harnett and colleagues discusses three diverse but inextricably interwoven perspectives (sociological, pharmacological and psychophysical) related to women as they age and their relationship to CIM.

Part II, 'CIM use and women's health issues', moves attention away from the women's life cycle to dissect the CIM and women's health field via three health conditions which all separately constitute significant health priority areas demanding attention with regards to wider populations. Nevertheless, in all cases, these conditions and the response to them are highlighted as raising specific (and sometimes unique) challenges for female sufferers with regards to treatment, coping and wider illness experience.

In Chapter 5, an international team of colleagues led by Schloss examine the current status and future potential of CIM for women's cancers. CIM in cancer care is a long-standing topic (e.g. Adams et al. 2005) that has rightly attracted much serious support and critique. As Schloss and her co-authors point out, while there remains only limited attention to women's cancer and CIM, these practices and products can play a major role in assisting the prevention, aid as an adjunct to treatment and increase the longevity of women diagnosed with cancer.

In Chapter 6, Adams and colleagues introduce new empirical findings regarding the use of CIM self-care among women with osteoarthritis and osteoporosis. As these scholars also explain, such a focus upon primarily patient-led activities, located in the community and undertaken while hidden from the gaze of conventional health care professionals (both in the hospital and formal primary health care setting) alerts us to some of the opportunities and challenges facing the CIM-conventional health care interface with regards to chronic illness more generally. Indeed, as Adams et al. suggest, to investigate CIM in isolation would be somewhat artificial and fail to adequately reflect the pluralistic reality of wider health care and health seeking behaviours (Sharma 2014), and it is imperative that empirical study engages the interface between CIM and other more conventional forms of health care – a theme revisited with regards to slightly different CIM-focused terrain in later chapters (e.g. Chapter 9) of this collection.

Part II is completed with an examination of CIM in relation to mental illness among women. In Chapter 7, McIntyre and colleagues describe CIM use by women for the specific treatment of depression and anxiety, and the evidence base for the most commonly used CIM for these conditions. These authors also introduce the integrative mental health care (IMHC) model which they argue is important for providing optimal mental health outcomes for women yet faces a number of barriers to successful implementation.

The final section, Part III, 'CIM, women and the health care system', widens the research gaze to explore a range of meta-issues relating to CIM – with a view to practice as well as use – which have a direct impact upon systems of health care (and the structured relationships therein) and/or disciplinary fields of enquiry. In Chapter 8, Andrews and DeMaio introduce a novel conceptual framework for investigating aspects of CIM use among female users. The authors claim that while qualitative studies tell us a lot about meaning and identity with respect to CIM, arguably, what has been largely missed to date is the immediacy of CIM – its happening in space and time materially, performatively and sensorily and this is no less the case for women's health and health care as for other topics regarding CIM. With reference to women's health, Andrews and DeMaio propose the adoption of non-representational theory (NRT) in qualitative research on CIM which can help address these neglects. The chapter closes with some thoughts on methodological challenges and more broadly on how NRT might be suitable for researching social intersectionality – such as gender – and the particular situations and challenges experienced by specific groups such as women.

In Chapter 9, Steel and colleagues explore the interface between maternity care providers and CIM. Overviewing a proposed paradigm first introduced by Davis-Floyd (2001), these authors explore the approaches of different maternity care providers and how they may influence their relationship to CIM – a pertinent issue given the substantial interest and use in CIM among pregnant women in contemporary maternity care as identified in Chapter 2 of this collection.

Chapter 10 draws upon two ad-hoc and somewhat small but nevertheless crucial bodies of literature within the CIM field – that detailing the (gender) workforce characteristics of CIM practitioners and that exploring the relationship between CIM practice and gender – to overview the current potential and future prospect of CIM to offer a feminist, female-orientated approach to health and health care. As Adams and colleagues suggest, such a potential remains contested and challenged by a number of contemporary circumstances facing CIM in late modern societies. It is interesting to note the majority of scholarship on the relationship between CIM practice/practitioners and gender was initiated a few years ago and, as with the vast majority of CIM sub-field topics, this remains an area in need of further in-depth fieldwork and analyses.

To close the collection, in Chapter 11, Leach and colleagues introduce the notion of a model of care – an overarching design for the provision of a particular type of health care service – to help describe a disconnect between women's health care needs and the dominant biomedical model of health care and to explore the current and possible future role CIM plays in addressing these needs.

Notwithstanding the now well-versed limitations of approaching and investigating CIM as an homogeneous field, and similarly of not acknowledging the complexities and variations of women's health and health care experiences and needs, it is hoped that this collection will act as a springboard for many, by helping introduce what, for them, may be new substantive topics, issues and challenges relating to CIM and women's health. Equally of importance, it is envisaged that this book will attract a wider audience beyond those specialising in CIM practice and research – the interface and relationship between gender and CIM can and should continue to constitute a rich source of innovation and reflection for all looking to provide, manage and ultimately understand women's health and health care.

# References

Adams, J., Andrews, G., Barnes, J., Broom, A. and Magin, P. (eds) (2012) *Traditional, Complementary and Integrative Medicine: An International Reader*, Basingstoke: Palgrave Macmillan.

Adams, J., Easthope, G. and Sibbritt, D. (2003a) 'Exploring the relationship between women's health and the use of complementary and alternative medicine', *Complementary Therapies in Medicine*, 11: 156–158.

Adams, J., Frawley, J., Steel, A., Broom, A. and Sibbritt, D. (2015) 'Use of pharmacological and non-pharmacological pain management techniques and their relationship to maternal and infant birth outcomes: Examination of a nationally representative sample of 1835 pregnant women', *Midwifery*, 31(4): 458–463.

Adams, J., Sibbritt, D., Easthope, G. and Young, A. (2003b) 'A profile of women who consult alternative health practitioners in Australia', *Medical Journal of Australia*, 179: 297–300.

Adams, J., Sibbritt, D. and Young, A. (2005) 'Naturopathy/herbalism consultations by mid-aged Australian women who have cancer', *European Journal of Cancer Care*, 14: 443–447.

Adams, J. and Tovey, P. (eds) (2008) *Complementary and Alternative Medicine in Nursing and Midwifery: Towards a Critical Social Science*, London: Routledge.

Bishop, F. and Lewith, G. (2010) 'Who uses CAM? A narrative review of demographic characteristics and health factors associated with CAM use', *Evidence-based Complementary and Alternative Medicine*, 7(1): 11–28.

Bishop, F., Northstone, K., Green, J. and Thompson, E. (2011) 'The use of complementary and alternative medicine in pregnancy: Data from the AVON Longitudinal Study of Parents and Children (ALSPAC)', *Complementary Therapies in Medicine*, 19(6): 303–310.

Davis-Floyd, R. (2001) 'The technocratic, humanistic, and holistic paradigms of childbirth', *International Journal of Gynecology & Obstetrics*, 75(Suppl. 1): S5–S23.

Flesch, H. (2007) 'Silent voices: Women, complementary medicine, and the co-optation of change', *Complementary Therapies in Clinical Practice*, 13(3): 166–173.

Sharma, U. (2014) 'Medical pluralism and the future of CAM', in M. Kelner and B. Wellman (eds) *Complementary and Alternative Medicine: Challenge and Change*, Amsterdam: Harwood Academic.

Steel, A., Adams, J., Sibbritt, D., Broom, A., Gallois, C. and Frawley, J. (2012) 'Utilisation of complementary and alternative medicine (CAM) practitioners within midwifery care provision: Results from a nationally representative cohort study of 1,835 pregnant women', *BMC Pregnancy and Childbirth*, 12: 146.

Steel, A., Frawley, J., Adams, J., Sibbritt, D. and Broom, A. (2013) 'Primary health care, complementary and alternative medicine and women's health: A focus upon menopause', in J. Adams, P. Magin and A. Broom (eds) *Primary Health Care and Complementary and Integrative Medicine: Practice and Research*, London: Imperial College Press.

Zhang, Y., Leach, M., Hall, H., Sundberg, T., Ward, L., Sibbritt, D. and Adams, J. (2015) 'Differences between male and female consumers of complementary and alternative medicine in a national US population: A secondary analysis of 2012 NHIS data', *Evidence-based Complementary and Alternative Medicine*, doi:10.1155/2015/413173.

# Part I

# CIM use and women's life cycle

# 1 The role of complementary and integrative medicine within preconception care

## Contributing to an emerging research field

*Abigail Aiyepola, Amie Steel, Jane Frawley and Jon Adams*

## Introduction

The aim of this chapter is to position and overview the potential of complementary and integrative medicine (CIM) within the empirical study and conceptual approach to the field of preconception health and service delivery. The chapter opens with a consideration of the history and context of preconception care including the emphasis placed on preconception care in contemporary policy documents developed by international health agencies. The chapter then examines current advances in our empirical understanding of the impact of maternal preconception health status on women's and neonates' health outcomes. The chapter also explores current knowledge regarding CIM and maternal health, particularly in the context of preconception care, and closes with a consideration of some key areas requiring research attention to help ensure future health service delivery and policy is responsive to women's needs during the preconception period, particularly as they relate to CIM.

## Preconception care: history and context

Cultures throughout human history have emphasised the importance of women maintaining health and being healthy prior to pregnancy (Freda et al., 2006). In recent decades, increasing recognition of the fetal origins of adult disease (FOAD) has contributed to a paradigm shift in the scientific understanding of disease etiology (Barker et al., 1995; Delisle, 2002). Some factors contributing to this paradigm shift include rising incidences of preterm births (Blencowe et al., 2013), paediatric and adult chronic diseases (Gluckman et al., 2008; Shonkoff et al., 2012) and neurodevelopmental disorders such as autism (Kolevzon et al., 2007). In particular, the fetal environment has been found to impact the risk of developing chronic diseases such as obesity (Ehrenthal et al., 2013), diabetes and cardio-vascular disease (Le Clair et al., 2009), and cancer (Miligi et al., 2013) through epigenetic and other cellular responses to developmental exposures (Wang et al., 2013). A substantial proportion of FOAD research examining the impact of low birth weight (LBW) as a surrogate marker of poor fetal growth and nutrition (Calkins and Devaskar, 2011) has reported links between LBW and coronary artery disease (Barker, 1995; Rogers and Velten, 2011), hypertension (Vickers et al., 2000), obesity (Oken and Gillman, 2003) and insulin resistance (Yajnik, 2004).

Alongside the growing physiological understanding of FOAD, is a cultural shift within medicine towards prevention and wellness (Hood and Friend, 2011), which is manifest in the policies and strategies underpinning contemporary preconception care (Moos, 2003). Deeper scientific and social investigations into the determinants of health have also contributed to this shift, as evidenced by the recent surge in epigenetic research (Cameron et al., 2008; Knezovich and Ramsay, 2012; Steegers-Theunissen and Steegers, 2015) and increasing emphasis on the social determinants of health (Hogan et al., 2012; Livingood et al., 2010).

These changes in the conceptualisation of disease aetiology have facilitated the development of preconception care as a meaningful preventive measure for achieving positive pregnancy and birth outcomes, as well as the ongoing optimal health of the offspring. Preconception care is an approach to health promotion and preventive medicine focused on interventions that identify and modify biomedical, behavioural and social risks to a woman's health or pregnancy outcome (Posner et al., 2006). In 2005, the Centers for Disease Control and Prevention in the USA hosted a summit with 35 partner organisations to help identify, among other related issues, a number of defining characteristics of preconception care (ibid.). The summit determined that effective preconception care cannot be achieved via one sole visit with a health professional but is a 'continuum of care designed to meet the needs of a woman through the various stages of her reproductive life' (ibid.). The summit participants also agreed that preconception care was, at its core, a health promotion initiative with the primary goal being to promote maternal and child health throughout a woman's reproductive lifespan, and facilitate each woman to be healthy as she attempts to conceive (ibid.). The summit also posited that one core focus of preconception interventions is to reduce perinatal risk factors.

According to the summit participants, preconception care relates to care before pregnancy, whether it is a first pregnancy or between consecutive pregnancies. Moving beyond the broad pronouncement of the summit, the importance of this component of contemporary health care has been acknowledged by a range of international bodies and organisations representing and regulating health professionals as well as health policy-makers (Christiansen et al., 2012; Committee on Gynecologic Practice, 2005; Johnson et al., 2006; National Institute for Health and Care Excellence, 2011). However, a recent review of preconception policies in six European countries highlights the fragmented, inconsistent and ad-hoc nature of preconception care polices in this space for healthy women and men (Shawe et al., 2015).

*The impact of preconception health status on outcomes for women
and neonates*

Preconception care has received increased attention due to growing evidence that
maternal health prior to conception can directly affect the health of the mother and
the fetal environment during pregnancy (Committee on Gynecologic Practice,
2005). The majority of research attention in this area over the last 20 years has
been directed towards the benefits of folic acid supplementation in preventing birth
defects (Berry et al., 1999; Boyles et al., 2011; Khodr et al., 2014; Wilson et al.,
2003; Yi et al., 2011). Meanwhile, the broader preconception care research field
emphasises the impact of the fetal environment on adverse outcomes such as
miscarriage (Nielsen et al., 2006), stillbirth (Signorello et al., 2010), congenital
disorders (Shannon et al., 2013) and macrosomia (Strutz et al., 2012).

Maternal health behaviours that are important in the context of preconception
care include dietary choices, smoking, alcohol consumption and exposure to
communicable diseases (Chandranipapongse and Koren, 2013; Coonrod et al.,
2008; Goldenberg and Thompson, 2003; Ji et al., 1997; Kind et al., 2006; Lassi
et al., 2014; MacArthur et al., 2008). In terms of diet, nutritional balance can
influence ovarian physiology and embryo quality (Kind et al., 2006). Parental
smoking preconception has been linked to serious conditions such as cancer
(Ji et al., 1997; MacArthur et al., 2008) and congenial heart defects (Lassi et al.,
2014) whereas preconception alcohol intake has been found to lead to a possible
30 per cent increase in spontaneous abortion (ibid.). Infection can cause stillbirths
(Goldenberg and Thompson, 2003) and while not directly attributable to maternal
behaviour, preventable actions can be taken to reduce the risk of infection during
the preconception period (Chandranipapongse and Koren, 2013; Coonrod et al.,
2008).

Despite these and other contemporary findings highlighting the pressing need
for preconception care to be prioritised within the general population, very little
research attention has been committed to understanding the use of preconception
services by women with chronic health conditions – arguably the sub-population
with greatest need for preconception care in the community. A recent systematic
review with no date restrictions only identified 14 papers examining this topic
worldwide (Steel et al., 2015). The majority of papers identified in this 2015 review
target women with type 1 or 2 diabetes, and failed to examine women with other
significant health conditions, such as thyroid disorders and epilepsy (Johnson et
al., 2006). Based on the outcomes of the review, on average, one in five women
with chronic health conditions engage with preconception care, those women who
did access preconception care commonly experienced emotional distress as a result,
women's knowledge of preconception care tends to be deficient in a number of
areas (Steel et al., 2015).

A second review, examining women's and health professionals' attitudes to
preconception care delivery, with the vast majority of literature identified as
focused upon health professionals' attitudes (Steel et al., 2016), highlighted the
emotional complexity associated with child-bearing decisions and women's need

for better quality information to inform their decision-making with regards to the risks and benefits of related health behaviours. The importance placed on preconception care in policy planning has limited translation into community-based care, according to data from the health professionals included in this review – some clinicians provide preconception services as part of routine care while others only deliver it opportunistically (Christiansen et al., 2012). More concerning was the review finding that indicates insufficient ownership of the delivery of preconception care services among health professionals and a self-identified gap in clinicians' knowledge with regards to providing effective preconception support (Steel et al., 2016).

## Complementary and integrative medicine and maternal health

Complementary and integrative medicine (CIM) are used by women to support their health during pregnancy, birth and the postnatal period. Research reports up to 80 per cent of women consult with a CIM practitioner or use CIM products for pregnancy-related health conditions (Adams et al., 2009; Frawley et al., 2013; Steel et al., 2012). Additional research also describes women's use of CIM products and treatments during labour to assist with pain management (Steel et al., 2013b) as well as CIM practitioner use in women's intrapartum birth team (Steel et al., 2013c). Likewise, women report using CIM in the postnatal period to assist with insufficient lactation (Sim et al., 2013).

Despite the substantive advances in preconception care research in recent years and the role CIM is known to play in women's wider health and health care (Adams et al., 2003; Peng et al., 2014; Rayner et al., 2011) and maternity services (Adams et al., 2009), very little research effort has been assigned to understanding the potential significance of CIM within preconception care. This neglected research area requires urgent attention with a view to helping ensure women and their families, health practitioners and health policy-makers are appropriately informed of all behaviours, decision-making and clinical evidence base regarding this important life stage.

## Connecting preconception care and preventive healthcare through CIM

Preventive health care is one aspect of contemporary medicine considered to be practised by all medical providers (physicians) while also existing as a unique medical specialty in its own right (American College of Preventive Medicine, 2017). Preventive health care aims to protect, promote, and maintain health and well-being and to prevent disease, disability, and death in individuals, communities and defined populations (ibid.). Preventive health practitioners combine population-based public health skills, such as health promotion and public education, with knowledge of primary, secondary and tertiary prevention-oriented clinical practice (Hensrud, 2000a). In the United States, preventive medicine is medical specialty practised by physicians who have completed additional training in preventive health care (American College of Preventive Medicine, 2017). However, in line with the diversity of preventive health interventions in place within health systems throughout the world, preventive health care may be practised by health professionals from a range of occupations and found in primary, secondary or tertiary health settings in both developed, transitional and developing countries (Jekel et al., 2007).

In the preventive health care framework, preconception care focuses upon controlling modifiable risk factors to avert the occurrence of disease and, as such, falls within the category of primary prevention (ibid.). Primary preventive health care relies on a number of strategies in a clinical setting to achieve better health outcomes, including health risk assessment and patient counselling and education (Hensrud, 2000b). However, these interventions are under-utilised for numerous clinician, patient and health system-based reasons (Hensrud, 2000a) and current missed opportunities in disease prevention, including underusing high value interventions, such as preconception care, have been linked with substantive increases in the burden of certain diseases (Olsen et al., 2010).

Preventive healthcare is listed among the qualities commonly employed to characterise CIM (Foley and Steel, 2017). Other qualities, such as holism, are also featured among the characteristics of many complementary medicine systems of care (ibid.) and have been described by women as necessary ingredients within preconception service delivery (Steel et al., 2015). Preconception care also features strongly within the curriculum and textbooks of CIM practitioner training programmes (Wardle and Steel, 2010).

Based on preventive medicine research more generally, there are a number of characteristics of primary prevention programmes that equally apply to preconception care (Nation et al., 2003) and highlight the importance of considering CIM when developing preconception care interventions. First, a programme must be comprehensive, meaning it must address all determinants (e.g. socioeconomic status, health literacy) and risk factors (e.g. alcohol consumption, smoking, health status) which may impact on maternal and fetal outcomes (Nation et al., 2003). It is recommended this be achieved through both multiple interventions (i.e. several interventions addressing the targeted health behaviour) and multiple settings (i.e. engage the systems that have impact on the development of the targeted health behaviour). Given the prevalence of CIM use among women during their reproductive years (Adams et al., 2009; Rayner et al., 2011), it is worth exploring whether CIM practitioners can have a role to play in modifying any of a number of problematic health behaviours among women attempting to conceive.

Second, preconception care interventions should encompass active, skills-based learning to address determinants and develop new behaviours to replace targeted health behaviours (Nation et al., 2003). Recent workforce data suggests CIM practitioners may include group education in their occupational role (Steel et al., 2017b), which, when considered alongside the intersect between the paradigms of some CIM professions and public health (Wardle and Oberg, 2012), implies these practitioners may hold the potential at least, if not already playing a health promotion role in the community which could be a valuable asset in preconception interventions.

Third, women need sufficient exposure to the preconception care intervention for it to have an effect (Nation et al., 2003) which aligns with the attribute of preconception care as a 'continuum of care' as distinct from a stand-alone clinical appointment (Posner et al., 2006) and relates to the duration of clinical appointments. As previous research reports, general practitioners commonly identify time constraints as a barrier to engaging meaningfully with primary preventive healthcare in general (Mirand et al., 2003), and preconception care in particular (Mazza et al., 2013). In contrast, users of CIM frequently describe the extended consultation time afforded by a CIM practitioner as a positive attribute which attracts them to seeking and receiving CIM care (Foley and Steel, 2016).

In line with previous research examining the experience of women accessing preconception programmes (Steel et al., 2015; Steel et al., 2016), primary prevention interventions should also be appropriately timed, socio-culturally relevant and engage well-trained health professionals (Nation et al., 2003). The importance of these last three principles should not be underestimated. The socio-cultural relevance of preconception services, in particular, requires close attention in the context of CIM, given the prevailing trends in high use of CIM among women (Adams et al., 2009; Rayner et al., 2011) and the importance of socio-cultural factors in driving such CIM use (Bishop et al., 2007).

## A possible agenda for future preconception care and CIM research

Despite the potential alignment between preconception care service delivery and CIM, there remains a dearth of research examining the role, place, value and impact of CIM as part of preconception care. As such, the development of evidence-based CIM interventions in this particular area of women's health requires sustained focus and resources. A range of approaches well suited to expanding our contemporary empirical investigation of preconception care can be found within the broad field of health services research (HSR) defined as 'the critical, scientific study of health and health care issues with a focus ranging from international, national and regional populations through to smaller localised/specialised groupings and individuals' (Adams et al., 2012). The research agenda outlined below is not definitive but does provide one framework for future HSR exploration of the role and value of CIM within preconception care.

### The use of CIM by women intending to conceive

There is a wide knowledge gap in understanding the prevalence of CIM use among women attempting to conceive. Recent Australian data indicates CIM practitioners are involved in the care of women during the preconception period (Steel et al., 2017a). This research shows women who attempt to conceive are more likely to consult with a naturopath or an acupuncturist compared to women not planning a pregnancy. Women who consult with an acupuncturist during this period are more likely to have also visited a specialist doctor and to have previous fertility issues. whereas women who consult with a naturopath for their preconception care were more likely to have experienced premenstrual tension and less likely to have had a previous miscarriage (ibid.). This Australian research constitutes the first in-depth examination of the role CIM practitioners play in providing care during the preconception period, and given that this draws upon a secondary analysis of data collected for more general research questions, there is still a substantial amount of research needed before a clearer picture of the nature and prevalence of CIM use by women during the preconception period is available (Rayner et al., 2009; Steel et al., 2017a).

In the first instance, the current research provides valuable information on the role of CIM practitioners in providing health care during the preconception period, but this research has only been conducted in one country and additional similar studies are needed in other locations for a clearer international picture on this topic to emerge. Furthermore, the Australian data does not elucidate whether women are visiting CIM practitioner specifically for assistance with conception or to improve maternal and child health outcomes, or if they are motivated by other factors (Steel et al., 2013a), and while the research suggests women differentiate between types of CIM practitioners when choosing who to access for preconception care, the specific perspectives and motivations that are driving these discrete treatment choices are not clear and require closer examination.

Even less is known about the use of the specific CIM products used by women during preconception care, including the reasons that may be motivating their individual or combined use. Women's perception of the safety of specific CIM products and, particularly in the case of self-prescribed CIM, where and how they access information which informs their decision-making are areas that have attracted attention with regards to women's other health issues (Frawley et al., 2014; Murthy et al., 2014) and equally require closer attention with regards to women's preconception care.

We also require more clarity regarding the nature and characteristics of the specific women who choose to use CIM in the preconception period. In direct response, a number of key research questions need to be answered, including: What are the motivations behind women using CIM for preconception care? Are there specific antenatal conditions women are attempting to prevent? Are such, are women motivated for the purposes of their own health, the health of their offspring, or both? For women who use CIM for preconception care, what role does conventional health care also play in their preconception health plan? Where are women accessing information regarding CIM for preconception care? Are women more or less likely to use CIM during preconception care if they have a history of CIM use? It is important that these questions are not only explored across the general population but that any differences between subsets of the population and the choice of CIM and CIM practitioner used for preconception care also receive attention. It is possible there are variations in the patterns of and motivations for

CIM use regarding preconception care accessed by healthy women compared to women with health conditions which may not affect pregnancy, and also women with health conditions known to affect pregnancy. As such, the areas outlined above need to be separately examined within each of these discrete subpopulations.

## The safety and effectiveness of CIM products and treatments within preconception care

The CIM products and treatments used by women and their partners during the preconception period also need to be closely examined for both safety and effectiveness. While research regarding the safety of CIM products for maternal health often centres on the antenatal (Izzo et al., 2016) or postnatal (Budzynska et al., 2012) periods, there is growing evidence that preconception exposures to some CIM products can have an impact on pregnancy and birth outcomes for women and their offspring (Lassi et al., 2014). As such, the possible risks associated with CIM products in this regard should not be overlooked. The evaluation of CIM for safety needs to focus on specific products which may be used to improve fertility, promote a more optimal pregnancy state and produce healthier offspring. Safety research must also focus on specific products which may be used to address other common health complaints not normally linked to pregnancy outcomes but still requiring treatment during the preconception period.

Likewise, the efficacy of CIM products used as part of a preconception care plan also require significant attention encompassing evaluations of CIM products used by some women to improve female fertility and egg quality, address menstrual irregularities or other hormonal influences, and promote overall improved pregnancy outcomes. Enquiry in this sub-field also needs to extend to CIM products which may be used to improve male fertility to assist with a range of factors which have been identified to impact on pregnancy success (Frey et al., 2008). This focus aligns with a broader gap in preconception care research already identified by expert consensus – that preconception care for both men *and* women is important in improving pregnancy outcomes (ibid.; Temel et al., 2015) – and needs to be considered within the context of CIM.

## The approach of CIM practitioners to preconception care

Beyond CIM products, it is also important to understand the approach of CIM practitioners to preconception care and the degree to which CIM practitioners promote preconception care among their patients. There is a proposed alignment between the underpinning principles of many CIM professions and the core elements of preconception care. For example, the emphasis on preventive medicine and education of patients within naturopathy (Foley and Steel, 2017), coupled with the apparent role CIM practitioners occupy in maternity service provision (Steel et al., 2012) suggests this alignment may manifest in real-life health service delivery. However, this alignment of approach requires further evidence before it can be confirmed.

As mentioned earlier in this chapter, recent workforce data suggests CIM practitioners may include group education within their health care approach and occupy a health promotion role in their wider community (Steel et al., 2017b). While current evidence does not provide clarity on the topics and materials covered in such group education activities, one in two practitioners from this recent study did identify women's health as an area of special clinical interest (ibid.). Given these recent advances in understanding CIM practice, more details are needed about whether CIM practitioners provide individualised or group education about preconception care and if so, what information CIM practitioners prioritise on this topic, particularly given women's expressed need for better information to support their decision-making (Steel et al., 2016). An understanding of the treatments and practices CIM practitioners use in their practice and prescribe to their patients as part of a preconception care plan similarly requires investigation.

The degree to which CIM practitioners integrate with existing public health programmes and primary health services when providing preconception care services to women and their partners must also be explored. By extension, the CIM practitioners' self-perceived contribution to preconception care for women and their partners and in relation to other health providers requires examination. Indeed, acknowledging and appreciating the role and contribution of CIM practitioners are particularly important, given the apparent lack of clear ownership of preconception care among many conventional health professions (ibid.; Temel et al., 2015).

## Conclusion

In an era of preventive medicine and epigenetics, the importance of effective preconception care has never been greater. The delivery of meaningful preconception care undoubtedly requires the development of services which respond to the needs and preferences of women and their families. Given the continued presence of CIM within contemporary health care delivery, research which explores CIM within the context of preconception care deserves urgent attention. Without more detailed information on the reasons women use (or fail to use) CIM for preconception care; the safety and effectiveness of CIM in the preconception period; and the contribution of CIM practitioners supporting women's preparation for pregnancy, the consideration of future policy and health service interventions in this significant women's health topic will be limited in scope and, as a result, effect.

## References

Adams, J., Andrews, G., Barnes, J., Broom, A. and Magin, P. (eds) 2012. *Traditional, Complementary and Integrative Medicine: An International Reader*. London: Palgrave.
Adams, J., Easthope, G. and Sibbritt, D. 2003. Exploring the relationship between women's health and the use of complementary and alternative medicine. *Complementary Therapies in Clinical Practice*, 11, 156–158.

Adams, J., Lui, C.-W., Sibbritt, D., et al. 2009. Women's use of complementary and alternative medicine during pregnancy: A critical review of the literature. *Birth*, 36, 237–245.

American College of Preventive Medicine. 2017. *Preventive Medicine* [Online]. Available at: www.acpm.org/page/preventivemedicine (accessed 17 December 2017).

Barker, D., Gluckman, P. and Robinson, J. 1995. Conference report: Fetal origins of adult disease—report of the first international study group, Sydney, 29–30 October 1994. *Placenta*, 16, 317–320.

Barker, D. J. 1995. Fetal origins of coronary heart disease. *BMJ: British Medical Journal*, 311, 171.

Berry, R. J., Li, Z., Erickson, J. D., Li, S. et al. 1999. Prevention of neural-tube defects with folic acid in China. *New England Journal of Medicine*, 341, 1485–1490.

Bishop, F. L., Yardley, L. and Lewith, G. T. 2007. A systematic review of beliefs involved in the use of complementary and alternative medicine. *Journal of Health Psychology*, 12, 851–867.

Blencowe, H., Cousens, S., Chou, D. et al. 2013. Born too soon: The global epidemiology of 15 million preterm births. *Reproductive Health*, 10, S2.

Boyles, A., Ballard, J., Gorman, E. et al. 2011. Association between inhibited binding of folic acid to folate receptor – in maternal serum and folate-related birth defects in Norway. *Human Reproduction*, 26, 2232–2238.

Budzynska, K., Gardner, Z. E., Dugoua, J.-J., Low Dog, T. and Gardiner, P. 2012. Systematic review of breastfeeding and herbs. *Breastfeeding Medicine*, 7, 489–503.

Calkins, K. and Devaskar, S. U. 2011. Fetal origins of adult disease. *Current Problems in Pediatric and Adolescent Health Care*, 41, 158–176.

Cameron, N. M., Shahrokh, D., Del Corpo, A. et al. 2008. Epigenetic programming of phenotypic variations in reproductive strategies in the rat through maternal care. *Journal of Neuroendocrinology*, 20, 795–801.

Chandranipapongse, W. and Koren, G. 2013. Preconception counseling for preventable risks. *Canadian Family Physician*, 59, 737–739.

Christiansen, C., Chandra-Mouli, V., Ogbaselassie, L., Willumsen, J. and Mason, E. 2012. *Meeting to Develop a Global Consensus on Preconception Care to Reduce Maternal and Childhood Mortality and Morbidity*. Geneva: World Health Organization.

Committee on Gynecologic Practice 2005. The importance of preconception care in the continuum of women's health care. ACOG Committee Opinion. Available at: www.acog.org/Resources-And-Publications/Committee-Opinions/Committee-on-Gynecologic-Practice/The-Importance-of-Preconception-Care-in-the-Continuum-of-Womens-Health-Care

Coonrod, D. V., Jack, B. W., Boggess, K. A. et al. 2008. The clinical content of preconception care: Immunizations as part of preconception care. *American Journal of Obstetrics and Gynecology*, 199, S290–S295.

Delisle, H. 2002. Programming of chronic disease by impaired fetal nutrition, in *Evidence and Implications for Policy and Intervention Strategies*. Geneva: World Health Organization.

Ehrenthal, D. B., Maiden, K., Rao, A. et al. 2013. Independent relation of maternal prenatal factors to early childhood obesity in the offspring. *Obstetrics & Gynecology*, 121, 115–121. Available at: http://10.1097/AOG.0b013e318278f56a

Foley, H. and Steel, A. 2016. Patient perceptions of clinical care in complementary medicine: A systematic review of the consultation experience. *Patient Education and Counseling*, 100, 2.

Foley, H. and Steel, A. 2017. The nexus between patient-centered care and complementary medicine: Allies in the era of chronic disease? *The Journal of Alternative and Complementary Medicine*, 23, 158–163.

Frawley, J., Adams, J., Broom, A., Steel, A., Gallois, C. and Sibbritt, D. 2014. Majority of women are influenced by nonprofessional information sources when deciding to consult a complementary and alternative medicine practitioner during pregnancy. *The Journal of Alternative and Complementary Medicine*, 20, 571–577.

Frawley, J., Adams, J., Sibbritt, D., Steel, A., Broom, A. and Gallois, C. 2013. Prevalence and determinants of complementary and alternative medicine use during pregnancy: Results from a nationally representative sample of Australian pregnant women. *Australian and New Zealand Journal of Obstetrics and Gynaecology*, 53, 347–352.

Freda, M. C., Moos, M.-K. and Curtis, M. 2006. The history of preconception care: Evolving guidelines and standards. *Maternal and Child Health Journal*, 10, 43–52.

Frey, K. A., Navarro, S. M., Kotelchuck, M. and Lu, M. C. 2008. The clinical content of preconception care: Preconception care for men. *American Journal of Obstetrics and Gynecology*, 199, S389–S395.

Gluckman, P. D., Hanson, M. A., Cooper, C. and Thornburg, K. L. 2008. Effect of in utero and early-life conditions on adult health and disease. *New England Journal of Medicine*, 359, 61–73.

Goldenberg, R. L. and Thompson, C. 2003. The infectious origins of stillbirth. *American Journal of Obstetrics and Gynecology*, 189, 861–873.

Hensrud, D. D. 2000a. Clinical preventive medicine in primary care: Background and practice: 1. Rationale and current preventive practices, in *Mayo Clinic Proceedings*. Oxford: Elsevier, pp. 165–172.

Hensrud, D. D. 2000b. Clinical preventive medicine in primary care: Background and practice: 2. Delivering primary preventive services, in *Mayo Clinic Proceedings*. Oxford: Elsevier, pp. 255–264.

Hogan, V. K., Rowley, D., Bennett, T. and Taylor, K. D. 2012. Life course, social determinants, and health inequities: Toward a national plan for achieving health equity for African American infants—a concept paper. *Maternal and Child Health Journal*, 16, 1143–1150.

Hood, L. and Friend, S. H. 2011. Predictive, personalized, preventive, participatory (P4) cancer medicine. *Nature Reviews Clinical Oncology*, 8, 184–187.

Izzo, A. A., Hoon-Kim, S., Radhakrishnan, R. and Williamson, E. M. 2016. A critical approach to evaluating clinical efficacy, adverse events and drug interactions of herbal remedies. *Phytotherapy Research*, 30, 691–700.

Jekel, J. F., Katz, D. L., Elmore, J. G. and Wild, D. 2007. *Epidemiology, Biostatistics and Preventive Medicine*. Oxford: Elsevier Health Sciences.

Ji, B.-T., Shu, X.-O., Zheng, W. et al. 1997. Paternal cigarette smoking and the risk of childhood cancer among offspring of nonsmoking mothers. *Journal of the National Cancer Institute*, 89, 238–243.

Johnson, K., Posner, S. F., Biermann, J., Cordero, J. F. and Atrash, H. 2006. Recommendations to improve preconception health and health care – United States. *Morbidity and Mortality Weekly Report (MMWR)*, 55, 1–23.

Khodr, Z. G., Lupo, P. J., Agopian, A. et al. 2014. Preconceptional folic acid-containing supplement use in the national birth defects prevention study. *Birth Defects Research Part A: Clinical and Molecular Teratology*, 100(6), 472–482.

Kind, K. L., Moore, V. M. and Davies, M. J. 2006. Diet around conception and during pregnancy – effects on fetal and neonatal outcomes. *Reproductive BioMedicine Online*, 12, 532–541.

Knezovich, J. G. and Ramsay, M. 2012. The effect of preconception paternal alcohol exposure on epigenetic remodeling of the h19 and rasgrf1 imprinting control regions in mouse offspring. *Frontiers in Genetics*, 3, 1–10/

Kolevzon, A., Gross, R. and Reichenberg, A. 2007. Prenatal and perinatal risk factors for autism: A review and integration of findings. *Archives of Pediatrics and Adolescent Medicine*, 161, 326–333.

Lassi, Z. S., Imam, A. M., Dean, S. V. and Bhutta, Z. A. 2014. Preconception care: Caffeine, smoking, alcohol, drugs and other environmental chemical/radiation exposure. *Reproductive Health*, 11, S6.

Le Clair, C., Abbi, T., Sandhu, H. and Tappia, P. S. 2009. Impact of maternal undernutrition on diabetes and cardiovascular disease risk in adult offspring. *Canadian Journal of Physiology and Pharmacology*, 87, 161–179.

Livingood, W. C., Brady, C., Pierce, K. et al. 2010. Impact of pre-conception health care: Evaluation of a social determinants focused intervention. *Maternal and Child Health Journal*, 14, 382–391.

Macarthur, A. C., McBride, M. L., Spinelli, J. J. et al. 2008. Risk of childhood leukemia associated with parental smoking and alcohol consumption prior to conception and during pregnancy: The cross-Canada childhood leukemia study. *Cancer Causes and Control*, 19, 283–295.

Mazza, D., Chapman, A. and Michie, S. 2013. Barriers to the implementation of preconception care guidelines as perceived by general practitioners: A qualitative study. *BMC Health Services Research*, 13, 36.

Miligi, L., Benvenuti, A., Mattioli, S. et al. 2013. Risk of childhood leukaemia and non-Hodgkin's lymphoma after parental occupational exposure to solvents and other agents: The SETIL Study. *Occupational and Environmental Medicine*, 70, 648–655.

Mirand, A. L., Beehler, G. P., Kuo, C. L. and Mahoney, M. C. 2003. Explaining the de-prioritization of primary prevention: Physicians' perceptions of their role in the delivery of primary care. *BMC Public Health*, 3, 15.

Moos, M. K. 2003. Preconceptional wellness as a routine objective for women's health care: An integrative strategy. *Journal of Obstetric, Gynecologic, and Neonatal Nursing*, 32, 550–556.

Murthy, V., Sibbritt, D., Adams, J. et al. 2014. Self-prescribed complementary and alternative medicine use for back pain amongst a range of care options: Results from a nationally representative sample of 1310 women aged 60–65 years. *Complementary Therapies in Medicine*, 22, 133–140.

Nation, M., Crusto, C., Wandersman, A. et al. 2003. What works in prevention: Principles of effective prevention programs. *American Psychologist*, 58, 449.

National Institute for Health and Care Excellence. 2011. *Preconception Care* [Online]. Available at: www.nice.org.uk/guidance/qualitystandards/diabetesinadults/preconception care.jsp (accessed 15 August 2013).

Nielsen, A., Gerd Hannibal, C., Eriksen Lindekilde, B. et al. 2006. Maternal smoking predicts the risk of spontaneous abortion. *Acta Obstetricia et Gynecologica Scandinavica*, 85, 1057–1065.

Oken, E. and Gillman, M. W. 2003. Fetal origins of obesity. *Obesity*, 11, 496–506.

Olsen, L., Saunders, R. S. and Yong, P. L. 2010. *The Healthcare Imperative: Lowering Costs and Improving Outcomes: Workshop Series Summary*. Washington, DC: National Academies Press.

Peng, W., Adams, J., Sibbritt, D. W. and Frawley, J. E. 2014. Critical review of complementary and alternative medicine use in menopause: Focus on prevalence, motivation, decision-making, and communication. *Menopause*, 21, 536–548.

Posner, S. F., Johnson, K., Parker, C., Atrash, H. and Biermann, J. 2006. The national summit on preconception care: A summary of concepts and recommendations. *Maternal and Child Health Journal*, 10, 199–207.

Rayner, J.-A., McLachlan, H. L., Forster, D. A. and Cramer, R. 2009. Australian women's use of complementary and alternative medicines to enhance fertility: Exploring the experiences of women and practitioners. *BMC Complementary and Alterntive Medicine* [Online], 9.

Rayner, J.-A., Willis, K. and Burgess, R. 2011. Women's use of complementary and alternative medicine for fertility enhancement: A review of the literature. *The Journal of Alternative and Complementary Medicine*, 17, 685–690.

Rogers, L. K. and Velten, M. 2011. Maternal inflammation, growth retardation, and preterm birth: Insights into adult cardiovascular disease. *Life Ssciences*, 89, 417–421.

Shannon, G. D., Alberg, C., Nacul, L. and Pashayan, N. 2013. Preconception health care and congenital disorders: Mathematical modelling of the impact of a preconception care programme on congenital disorders. *British Journal of Obstetrics and Gynaecology*, 120, 555–567.

Shawe, J., Delbaere, I., Ekstrand, M. et al. 2015. Preconception care policy, guidelines, recommendations and services across six European countries: Belgium (Flanders), Denmark, Italy, the Netherlands, Sweden and the United Kingdom. *The European Journal of Contraception and Reproductive Health Care*, 20, 77–87.

Shonkoff, J.P., Garner, A.S., Committee on Psychosocial Aspects of Child and Family Health; Committee on Early Childhood, Adoption, and Dependent Care; Section on Developmental and Behavioral Pediatrics 2012. The lifelong effects of early childhood adversity and toxic stress. *Pediatrics*, 129, e232–e246.

Signorello, L. B., Mulvihill, J. J., Green, D. M. et al. 2010. Stillbirth and neonatal death in relation to radiation exposure before conception: A retrospective cohort study. *Lancet*, 376, 624–630.

Sim, T. F., Sherriff, J., Hattingh, H. L., Parsons, R. and Tee, L. B. 2013. The use of herbal medicines during breastfeeding: A population-based survey in Western Australia. *BMC Complementary and Alternative Medicine*, 13, 317.

Steegers-Theunissen, R. P. and Steegers, E. A. 2015. Embryonic health: New insights, health and personalised patient care. *Reproduction, Fertility and Development*, 27, 712–715.

Steel, A., Adams, J. and Sibbritt, D. 2017a. The characteristics of women who use complementary medicine while attempting to conceive: results from a nationally representative sample of 13,224 Australian women. *Women's Health Issues*, 27, 67–74.

Steel, A., Adams, J., Sibbritt, D. et al. 2012. Utilisation of complementary and alternative medicine (CAM) practitioners within maternity care provision: results from a nationally representative cohort study of 1,835 pregnant women. *BMC Pregnancy Childbirth* [Online], 12.

Steel, A., Adams, J., Sibbritt, D., et al. 2013a. Determinants of women consulting with a complementary and alternative medicine practitioner for pregnancy-related health conditions. *Women's Health*, 54, 127–144.

Steel, A., Adams, J., Sibbritt, D. et al. 2013b. Managing the pain of labour: Factors associated with the use of labour pain management for pregnant Australian women. *Health Expectations*, doi: 10.1111/hex.12155.

Steel, A., Frawley, J., Sibbritt, D. and Adams, J. 2013c. A preliminary profile of Australian women accessing doula care: Findings from the Australian Longitudinal Study on Women's Health. *Australian and New Zealand Journal of Obstetrics and Gynaecology*, 53, 589–592.

Steel, A., Leach, M., Wardle, J. et al. 2017b. The Australian Complementary Medicine workforce: A profile of 1,306 practitioners from the PRACI study. *The Journal of Alternative and Complementary Medicine*, in press.

Steel, A., Lucke, J. and Adams, J. 2015. The prevalence and nature of use of preconception services by women with chronic health conditions: An integrative review. *BMC Women's Health*, 15, doi: 10.1186/s12905-015-0165-6.

Steel, A., Lucke, J., Reid, R. and Adams, J. 2016. A systematic review of women's and health professionals' attitudes and experience of preconception care service delivery. *Family Practice*, in press.

Strutz, K. L., Richardson, L. J. and Hussey, J. M. 2012. Preconception health trajectories and birth weight in a national prospective cohort. *Journal of Adolescent Health*, 51, 629–636.

Temel, S., Van Voorst, S. F., De Jong-Potjer, L. C. et al. 2015. The Dutch national summit on preconception care: A summary of definitions, evidence and recommendations. *Journal of Community Genetics*, 6, 107.

Vickers, M. H., Breier, B. H., Cutfield, W. S. et al. 2000. Fetal origins of hyperphagia, obesity, and hypertension and postnatal amplification by hypercaloric nutrition. *American Journal of Physiology, Endocrinology and Metabolism*, 279, E83–E87.

Wang, G., Walker, S. O., Hong, X. et al. 2013. Epigenetics and early life origins of chronic noncommunicable diseases. *Journal of Adolescent Health*, 52, S14–S21.

Wardle, J. and Oberg, E. 2012. The intersecting paradigms of naturopathic medicine and public health: Opportunities for naturopathic medicine. *Journal of Alternative and Complementary Medicine*, 17, 1079–1084.

Wardle, J. and Steel, A. 2010. Fertility, preconception care and pregnancy, in J. Sarris and J. Wardle (eds) *Clinical Naturopathy: An Evidence-Based Guide to Practice*. Chatswood: Elsevier.

Wilson, R., Davies, G., Desilets, V. et al. 2003. The use of folic acid for the prevention of neural tube defects and other congenital anomalies. *Journal of Obstetrics and Gynaecology Canada, JOGC; Journal d'obstétrique et gynécologie du Canada: JOGC*, 25, 959–973.

Yajnik, C. 2004. Early life origins of insulin resistance and type 2 diabetes in India and other Asian countries. *The Journal of Nutrition*, 134, 205–210.

Yi, Y., Lindemann, M., Colligs, A. and Snowball, C. 2011. Economic burden of neural tube defects and impact of prevention with folic acid: A literature review. *European Journal of Pediatrics*, 170, 1391–1400.

# 2 Complementary and integrative medicine use in pregnancy

## Focus upon contemporary analysis of self-prescribed treatment among Australian women

*Jane Frawley, Amie Steel, Matthew Leach, Abigail Aiyepola and Jon Adams*

## Introduction

Global interest in complementary and integrative medicine (CIM) has risen exponentially over recent decades, with recent research from a number of countries indicating that this interest in CIM may also extend to pregnancy (Frawley et al. 2013). Two recent literature reviews have highlighted the growing research interest and widespread use of CIM during pregnancy (Adams et al. 2009; Hall et al. 2011) and this chapter draws upon the findings of these two reviews and more recent literature as well as new analyses from contemporary fieldwork to examine the current opportunities and challenges of CIM use, specifically self-prescribed CIM, among pregnant women.

## CIM use during pregnancy: an overview of the current literature

International estimates of CIM use during pregnancy vary considerably. However, CIM use appears to be increasing with research across a number of countries identifying up to 87 per cent of pregnant women are using some form of CIM (Hall and Jolly 2014; Sibbritt et al. 2014) and despite some regional differences, women who use CIM during pregnancy generally have a higher level of education compared to women who do not use CIM (Adams et al. 2011; Bishop et al. 2011; Gaffney and Smith 2004a; Kennedy et al. 2013; Strouss et al. 2014). Research demonstrates that women who use CIM during pregnancy are more likely to have used CIM prior to pregnancy, possibly indicating that women are more confident in using certain CIM remedies and methods familiar to them (Gaffney and Smith 2004a; Hope-Allan et al. 2004; Kalder et al. 2011; Lapi et al. 2010).

Women who use CIM during pregnancy are also increasingly likely to report more physical symptoms than women who do not (Skouteris et al. 2008). Further to this, Adams et al. (2011) found that women who used vitamins and minerals during pregnancy had poorer general health and thus had considerably lower Short Form-36 (SF-36) physical component scores than non-users. Studies have shown that the use of CIM in pregnancy is significantly associated with other pregnancy-related health concerns such as fatigue, urinary tract infection, nausea and vomiting, and preparation for labour (Adams et al. 2009; Adams et al. 2011). Further research has found that pregnant women use CIM for specific conditions such as back pain or back ache, neck pain, labour preparation, coughs and colds, and indigestion (Frawley et al. 2013; Skouteris et al. 2008).

Use of CIM during pregnancy appears to be mediated, at least in part, by a desire for a natural approach that is nontoxic and effective (Holst et al. 2009; Westfall 2003). Many women believe that CIM is as safe as conventional medicine during pregnancy (Lapi et al. 2010; Nordeng and Havnen 2004); with some women believing it is less harmful (Bercaw et al. 2010; Holst et al. 2009; Lapi et al. 2010; Westfall 2003).

Women often cite concern related to loss of control, and the desire for a holistic approach as reasons for using CIM during pregnancy. Childbirth is viewed as a stressful experience for some women that evokes feelings of vulnerability and loss of control (Mitchell 2010); CIM may offer a sense of control and choice by enabling women to make some maternity health care decisions themselves (Gaffney and Smith 2004b; Warriner et al. 2014).

Women use various professional and non-professional sources of information when looking for guidance about CIM use during pregnancy. Research has identified that up to 33 per cent of pregnant women access conventional practitioners, such as obstetricians, doctors, nurses, midwives and pharmacists, for information on CIM at this time (Cagayan and Oras 2010; Forster et al. 2006; Frawley et al. 2013; Hollyer et al. 2002; Holst et al. 2009; Lapi et al. 2010; Nordeng and Havnen 2004; Westfall 2003). Up to 38 per cent of pregnant women also consult CIM practitioners for advice on CIM use (Forster et al. 2006; Hepner et al. 2002; Hollyer et al. 2002; Holst et al. 2009 Lapi et al. 2010; Nordeng and Havnen 2004; Pettigrew et al. 2004).

Research demonstrates that up to 71 per cent of women access non-professional sources of information regarding CIM use during pregnancy, which includes relying on their own experience, and attaining advice from friends, family, the media, books, magazines, the Internet and health food shops (Cagayan and Oras 2010; Forster et al. 2006; Frawley et al. 2015; Hepner et al. 2002; Hollyer et al. 2002; Holst et al. 2009a; Lapi et al. 2010; Maats and Crowther 2002; Nordeng and Havnen 2004; Pettigrew et al. 2004; Westfall 2003). 'Friends and family' are consistently reported as popular sources of information on CIM use during pregnancy, with between 14 per cent and 61.8 per cent of women seeking their advice (Cagayan and Oras 2010; Forster et al. 2006; Hepner et al. 2002; Hollyer et al. 2002; Holst et al. 2009; Lapi et al. 2010; Maats and Crowther 2002; Nordeng and Havnen 2004; Pettigrew et al. 2004; Westfall 2003).

Recent research suggests up to 75 per cent of women fail to disclose their use of CIM to maternity care providers (Bercaw et al. 2010; Holst et al. 2009; Strouss et al. 2014). Rates of disclosure vary considerably between studies. A US study found as few as 1 per cent of participants disclosed their use of CIM to a maternity care professional in 2006, compared to 50 per cent in 2013 (Strouss et al. 2014). Another study found that although 33 per cent of women did not disclose their CIM use during pregnancy to their doctor or midwife, 81.3 per cent of study participants had not been asked about their CIM use (Hall and Jolly 2014). Some women appear to be reluctant to disclose their use of CIM during this time due to fear of encountering negative attitudes and feeling chastised by their medical provider (Holst et al. 2009), whereas other women may be more likely to disclose their use of CIM if asked (Hall and Jolly 2014).

## Women's self-prescription of CIM products during pregnancy

The self-prescribing of CIM products is prevalent during pregnancy, with studies revealing between 22 per cent and 71 per cent of women prescribe products for themselves (Forster et al. 2006; Frawley et al. 2015; Holst et al. 2009; Nordeng and Havnen 2004; Westfall 2003). Most of the data collected on women's self-prescription of CIM products during pregnancy has been in relation to herbal medicines, possibly due to particular concerns about the potential teratogenic nature of some herbal medicines (Frawley et al. 2015).

It appears that the rate of herbal medicine self-prescription during pregnancy may vary for different herbs. Forster et al. (2006) asked 588 pregnant women to identify who prescribed the herbal medicines they were using, namely, raspberry leaf, ginger, chamomile, cranberry juice, echinacea, evening primrose oil, digestive bitters and Chinese herbs. The self-prescription of herbal medicines (other than Chinese herbal medicine) ranged from 33–71 per cent, with higher rates noted for ginger (42 per cent), chamomile (71 per cent), cranberry juice (63 per cent) and echinacea (59 per cent), as compared to recommendations by a naturopath, friend, family member or doctor. It may be possible that herbs in common use are considered to be more innocuous than unfamiliar herbs and are therefore thought to be safe during pregnancy. A more recent study has provided further evidence that the self-prescription of herbal medicine during pregnancy is high throughout many regions of the world (Kennedy et al. 2013). Across the six regions surveyed, namely Western Europe (n = 3,201), Northern Europe (n = 2,820), Eastern Europe (n = 2,342), North America (n = 533), South America (n = 346) and Australia (n = 217), researchers found that herbal medicine self-prescription ranged from 22.5 per cent in Australia to 31.9 per cent in Northern Europe.

Even though the use of some CIM services during pregnancy may be innocuous, the ingestion of CIM products for which there is little evidence of safety is more concerning. Preliminary data does suggest some CIM commonly used in pregnancy, such as ginger, may be safe for use by pregnant women (Borelli et al. 2005). However, a wider examination of commonly used herbal medicines high-lights an absence of comprehensive safety data which requires well-trained health professionals to provide appropriate advice and guidance to women using herbal medicines during pregnancy (Cuzzolin and Benoni 2009).

While some of these CIM may be appropriate if used under supervision by a qualified practitioner, there are concerns if these products are self-prescribed without input from a health care professional. These concerns were highlighted in a recent survey of US obstetric-gynecology patients, which found most women do not refer to their health care practitioner prior to commencing CIM (Furlow et al. 2008). Similarly, women's disclosure of CIM use to conventional health practitioners is often sub-optimal (Harrigan 2011; Strouss et al. 2014).

## Analyses of self-prescribed CIM product use among a nationally representative sample of 1,835 Australian women

Although a growing number of studies have examined the prevalence of CIM use in pregnancy (Adams et al. 2009; Hall et al. 2011), few have provided in-depth, exclusive analysis of self-prescribed CIM product use in this population. Furthermore, of those papers that have reported on self-prescription of CIM, most have been concerned with the use of herbal medicine only (Forster et al. 2006; Holst et al. 2009; Nordeng and Havnen 2004; Westfall 2003). In the interest of improving maternal and neonatal outcomes, it is important to determine the frequency with which women self-prescribe different CIM products during pregnancy. This information will be valuable in informing the development of strategies to improve patient/health professional communication, as well as patient education regarding CIM product use during pregnancy. Accordingly, this chapter now turns attention to the analyses and findings from a contemporary study investigating the prescription and self-prescription of CIM products during pregnancy in a nationally representative sample of pregnant Australian women.

### *Methods*

#### *Study design*

A secondary analysis of data collected from the Australian Longitudinal Study on Women's Health (ALSWH) was undertaken. The ALSWH – a 20-year longitudinal study of health and health service use that commenced in 1996 – aims to examine the health and well-being of Australian women across three age groups (i.e. 18–23 years, 45–50 years and 70–75 years). These women, who were randomly selected from the Medicare Australia database, were shown to be broadly representative of the national Australian population of women in the three target age groups (Brown et al. 1999). A more detailed description of the ALSWH is reported elsewhere (ibid.).

#### *Procedure*

The study sample was obtained via a sub-study of ALSWH participants. In the most recent (2009) survey of the youngest cohort (i.e. survey 5 of 8,199 women then aged 31–36 years), 2,316 women indicated that they were currently pregnant or had recently given birth. These women were invited to participate in the 2010 sub-study to investigate their use of complementary medicine for pregnancy health conditions during their most recent pregnancy; details of this sample are described elsewhere in more detail (Frawley et al. 2015). The questionnaire was mailed to 2,316 women, and return of the completed questionnaire implied consent.

*Survey*

The self-administered, paper-based questionnaire comprised 85 items, which included a combination of closed and open-ended questions. Items related to three key areas: (1) participant demographics; (2) health status; and (3) health service use. In relation to the latter, women were asked if they had used any CIM products (e.g. herbal tincture/tablets/pills, herbal tea, vitamins/minerals, aromatherapy oils, homeopathy, or flower essences) during their pregnancy for pregnancy-related health conditions. Women were also asked to designate if the products were self-prescribed or prescribed by a practitioner. If women answered yes to the latter, they were asked if the prescribing practitioner was a conventional medical practitioner (e.g. general practitioner, obstetrician, midwife) or a complementary medicine practitioner (not specified).

*Statistical analysis*

Data on prescription were re-coded to produce four variables: (1) self-prescribed; (2) medical practitioner prescribed; (3) CIM practitioner prescribed; and (4) not used. Descriptive statistics (e.g. frequency distributions) were used to depict the percentage of women who used CIM products during pregnancy, the number who self-prescribed these medicines, and the conventional and complementary medicine practitioners who prescribed these medicines. All analyses were conducted using STATA 11.2 (StataCorp LP, Texas, US).

*Ethics*

Ethics approval for this sub-study was obtained from the Human Research Ethics Committees of the University of Newcastle (#H-2010_0031), University of Queensland (#2010000411) and the University of Technology Sydney (#2011-174N).

**Results**

A total of 2,316 women were invited to participate in the sub-study. Some 1,835 women responded to the survey, providing a response rate of 79.2 per cent. Overall, 3.2 per cent of respondents self-prescribed a herbal medicine product (i.e. tincture, tablets or pills) and 8 per cent were prescribed a herbal product by a practitioner (Table 2.1). A total of 25.1 per cent of women self-prescribed a herbal tea while 5.3 per cent were prescribed this product by a practitioner. For vitamins/minerals,

*Table 2.1* The self-prescription of CIM products during pregnancy for pregnancy-related health conditions

| | Self-prescribed n (%) | | Practitioner prescribed n (%) | | Did not use n (%) | |
|---|---|---|---|---|---|---|
| Herbal medicine (tincture, tablets, pills, etc.) | 55 | (3.2) | 135 | (8.0) | 1,503 | (88.8) |
| Herbal tea | 431 | (25.1) | 91 | (5.3) | 1,193 | (69.6) |
| Vitamins/minerals | 802 | (41.1) | 947 | (48.6) | 200 | (10.3) |
| Aromatherapy oils | 131 | (7.8) | 24 | (1.4) | 1,521 | (90.8) |
| Homeopathy | 22 | (1.4) | 53 | (3.2) | 1,599 | (95.4) |
| Flower essences | 79 | (4.8) | 35 | (2.1) | 1,550 | (93.1) |

*Table 2.2* Self-prescribed, medical practitioner and CIM practitioner prescribed CIM products for pregnancy-related health conditions

| | Self-prescribed n (%) | | Medical practitioner prescribed n (%) | | CIM practitioner prescribed n (%) | |
|---|---|---|---|---|---|---|
| Herbal medicine (tincture, tablets, pills, etc.) | 55 | (28.2) | 68 | (34.9) | 72 | (36.9) |
| Herbal tea | 431 | (81.6) | 57 | (10.8) | 40 | (7.6) |
| Vitamins/minerals | 802 | (45.2) | 903 | (50.9) | 69 | (3.9) |
| Aromatherapy oils | 131 | (84.0) | 12 | (7.7) | 13 | (8.3) |
| Homeopathy | 22 | (28.9) | 11 | (14.5) | 43 | (56.6) |
| Flower essences | 79 | (68.1) | 11 | (9.5) | 26 | (22.4) |

41.1 per cent self-prescribed these products and 48.6 per cent were prescribed by a practitioner. Women also self-prescribed aromatherapy oils (7.8 per cent vs. 1.4 per cent practitioner-prescribed), homeopathy (1.4 per cent vs. 3.2 per cent practitioner-prescribed) and flower essences (4.8 per cent vs. 2.1 per cent practitioner-prescribed).

Of the women who used CIM products during pregnancy for pregnancy-related health issues, 84 per cent self-prescribed aromatherapy oils, 81.6 per cent herbal teas, 45.2 per cent vitamin/mineral supplements, 28.2 per cent herbal tinctures/tablets/pills, and 28.9 per cent homeopathic medicines (Table 2.2).

Among the women using CIM during pregnancy, 71.8 per cent of herbal medicines were practitioner-prescribed, followed by 71.1 per cent of homeopathic medicines, 54.8 per cent of vitamin/mineral supplements, 31.9 per cent of flower essences, 18.4 per cent of herbal teas and 16.0 per cent of aromatherapy oils (Table 2.2). The products most likely to be prescribed by CIM practitioners were homeopathic medicines and flower essences. CIM products most likely to be prescribed by conventional medical practitioners were vitamin/mineral supplements and herbal teas.

# Discussion

Our study set out to determine the extent to which women self-prescribe CIM products during pregnancy in a nationally representative sample of 1,835 young Australian pregnant women. The use of vitamin and mineral supplementation during pregnancy was found to be common, with half of the women identifying conventional medical practitioners as prescribers of these supplements. The recommendation of these products by medical practitioners is not surprising given the level of acceptance by the medical community of the role of some nutrients in reducing the risk of certain conditions, including the use of folate to decrease the likelihood of neural tube defects (Wallingford et al. 2013), and iron to protect against iron deficiency anaemia in women at risk (Imdad and Bhutta 2012). Previous Australian research corroborates the popularity of vitamin and mineral supplementation during pregnancy (Forster et al. 2009; Gaffney and Smith 2004a; Maats and Crowther 2002; Skouteris et al. 2008) with one study revealing that 91 per cent of women take a vitamin or mineral supplement during pregnancy, of which folic acid and iron were the most frequently reported (Forster et al. 2009).

While fewer women from our study used herbal medicines during pregnancy than nutrient supplements, self-prescription rates were relatively high for herbal medicines (i.e. 82 per cent of herbal teas and 28 per cent of herbal tinctures/tablets/pills). International studies have presented more conservative estimates of self-prescribed herbal medicine use in pregnancy. In a multi-national survey involving 9,459 women from 23 countries, researchers found herbal medicine self-prescription ranged from 22.5 per cent in Australia to 31.9 per cent in Northern Europe (Kennedy et al. 2013). Similarly, a survey of 400 Norwegian women found 22.9 per cent of those who used herbal medicine during pregnancy had initiated this use themselves (Nordeng and Havnen 2004). Further, focus groups involving 27 Canadian pregnant women found 32 per cent of women were guided by prior knowledge and 12 per cent by intuition when self-prescribing herbal medicine products for use during pregnancy (Westfall 2003).

An additional layer of complexity in relation to the high level of use of self-prescribed herbal medicines in pregnancy is the discrepancy in the regulation of herbal medicines compared with herbal teas in Australia. To elaborate, herbal medicines are regulated by the Therapeutic Goods Administration (TGA 2014) and as such, health claims, manufacturing processes and product information on labels of herbal medicines are carefully controlled. By contrast, herbal teas are regulated as a food product through Food Standards Australia and New Zealand, which is focused primarily on food safety and contamination with little attention to health claims and lower requirements for ingredient labelling (FSANZ 2013). The outcome of these different levels of regulation is that women using herbal teas during pregnancy may be at risk of unknowingly using a species of plant that is unsafe in pregnancy.

Other plant-based products such as aromatherapy oils are also commonly used during pregnancy (Bastard and Tiran 2006; Gaffney and Smith 2004a; Skouteris et al. 2008), typically for conditions such as nausea, urinary tract infection, headaches, insomnia and allergies (Adams et al. 2009; Sibbritt et al. 2014). Some authors, however, have raised the concern that aromatherapy oils may be harmful to a developing foetus with some oils possessing abortifacient properties (Watt and Janca 2008). While commonly used aromatherapy oil could be considered to have a low associated risk when used as recommended, their safety during pregnancy has not been demonstrated (Lis-Balchin 1999). These risks may be associated with direct risks of ingestion or application at high concentrations, or they may be linked to indirect risks associated with product adulteration (ibid.). Given the high-level (84 per cent) of self-prescribed aromatherapy use in our sample, the ease of access to essential oils in Australia, and aforementioned concerns about the potential risks of some essential oils, it is possible that a proportion of women may be putting themselves or their unborn baby at risk of harm, unintentionally.

The high rate of self-prescription of complementary medicines among pregnant women may in part be explained by the accessibility of CIM products. Products such as multivitamins, folic acid, calcium, vitamin C, vitamin B6 and vitamin A (retinol) are all readily available in pharmacies and retail outlets (McKenna and McIntyre 2006). Equally, herbal medicines such as peppermint, cranberry, and St. John's wort are available over the counter and are used by pregnant women despite the absence of clear safety data (ibid.). Some concerns have been raised regarding the accessibility of over-the-counter CIM products with a recent Australian government review examining the appropriateness of CIM retail product sales through pharmacies (SANOFI 2016). While the Therapeutic Goods Administration in Australia enforces internationally recognised standards of manufacturing and labelling (Therapeutic Goods Administration 2016), the effectiveness of these standards relies heavily on consumer health literacy (Carbone and Zoellner 2012). However, the wide availability of CIM products is expected to continue for the foreseeable future, potentially exposing pregnant women who choose to self-prescribe these products to the risks associated with unsupervised use.

The very nature of self-prescription means that women do not usually seek advice before commencing use, leading to concerns about adequate monitoring as well as direct and indirect risks. Direct risk relates to the risk of the medications themselves, such as teratogenic and abortifacient effects (Sibbritt et al. 2014; Watt and Janca 2008). Indirect risk refers to the risk associated with poor diagnosis and ineffectual, delayed or incorrect treatment. These risks are of serious concern as delayed and/or unsuccessful treatment of a pregnancy-related health concern may escalate the health problem, and in some cases, may adversely affect the health of the baby and mother (Sibbritt et al. 2014).

An example of where indirect risks may be of concern for pregnant women is the high level of use of self-prescribed flower essences. Flower essences are natural remedies that are purported to assist individuals to balance emotional states (Waterworth 2011). There is no known clinical research to verify the safety and/or efficacy of flower essences for pregnancy-related health conditions and observational data suggests that women using flower essences for pregnancy-related health conditions are three times more likely to experience emotional distress associated with labour (Steel et al. 2014). The prevalence of antenatal depression and anxiety is substantial (Bennett et al. 2004) and both illnesses are known precursors to postnatal depression (Verreault et al. 2014) – a condition associated with adverse outcomes for both mother and baby (O'Hara and McCabe 2013). It is possible that women who are self-prescribing flower essences have antenatal depression or anxiety, either diagnosed or undiagnosed, and are using flower essences to manage their mental health. Should this be the case, these women and their offspring are potentially exposed to the indirect risk (Wardle and Seely 2007) of using an ineffectual treatment to address an important maternal and infant health issue. Perhaps in contrast to the past, women in contemporary society are more likely to make health care decisions for themselves (Passmore 2008). Access to multiple sources of health and medical information via various media channels, including the Internet, have made it increasingly easy for women to determine their health care needs and navigate various treatment options. An enormous volume of information is available that focuses on notions such as "wellness" or "well-being", and natural and holistic health care; concepts that are known to be important to women who use CIM during pregnancy (Warriner et al. 2014).

A recent study found that women associate self-management techniques with the idea of well-being (McMahon et al. 2014) and this may, at least in part, underpin the use and self-prescription of CIM products during pregnancy. Additionally, our study found conventional medical practitioners prescribed a reasonable proportion of CIM products. This study found that of the women who used herbal medicine tinctures, tablets or pills during pregnancy, a medical doctor, obstetrician or mid-wife prescribed 35 per cent of these products. Conventional medical practitioners prescribed 51 per cent of the vitamins and minerals used by pregnant women, 15 per cent of homeopathy products and 10 per cent of flower essences. This suggests that there is at least some level of acceptance of CIM products among these health care providers. This claim is consistent with previous reports that show many general practitioners, obstetricians, midwives and pharmacists have positive views concerning CIM use (Gaffney and Smith 2004b).

Despite the positive views of CIM held by some conventional health care providers, research still shows that most women do not disclose their use of CIM during pregnancy to these health care professionals (Harrigan 2011). Some women appear reluctant to disclose their use of CIM during pregnancy due to fear of encountering negative attitudes and feeling chastised (Holst et al. 2009), whereas other women simply state that they were not asked (Hall and Jolly 2014). Lack of disclosure may compound any problems associated with the self-prescription of CIM products during pregnancy.

There are some limitations to our study that are worth noting. First, the survey was self-administered, relying on a woman's memory of CIM use during pregnancy; this may have introduced recall bias and limited the strength of the findings. Second, the study was conducted in women aged 31–36 years and there-fore did not include women over the age of 36 years; a demographic where fertility rates are increasing (ABS 2014). Finally, women were asked to 'mark all that apply' in relation to who prescribed their CIM products, making a comparative analysis impossible. Despite these limitations, the use of a sizeable, well-established, nationally representative data set of pregnant women provides valuable information in relation to prescribing patterns, including the self-prescription of CIM during pregnancy.

## Conclusion

Our findings suggest that Australian women frequently self-prescribe CIM products during pregnancy. While many of these products may indeed be harmless, the safety of some of these products has not been established in pregnancy. Thus, it is important for health care providers to facilitate an open and frank conversation with women in relation to CIM use during pregnancy to ascertain if any unsafe CIM products are being used; this is critical to safeguarding the mother and unborn baby from potential harm.

## Acknowledgements

The Australian Longitudinal Study on Women's Health, which was conceived and developed by groups of interdisciplinary researchers at the University of Queensland, University of Newcastle and University of Queensland, is funded by the Australian Department of Health and Ageing. We thank all participants for their valuable contribution to the study described in this chapter. We also thank the NHMRC for funding Professor Jon Adams while working on this project via an NHMRC Career Development Fellowship as well as the ARC for funding this project via a Discovery Project Grant (DP1094765).

## References

ABS (Australian Bureau of Statistics). (2014) 3301.0 – Births, Australia, 2013. Canberra, Australia: ABS. Available at: www.abs.gov.au/ausstats/abs@.nsf/mf/3301.0

Adams, J., Andrews, G., Barnes, J., Broom, A. and Magin, P. (2012) *Traditional, Complementary and Integrative Medicine: An International Reader*. Basingstoke: Palgrave Macmillan.

Adams, J., Easthope, G. and Sibbritt, D. (2003) 'Exploring the relationship between women's health and the use of complementary and alternative medicine', *Complementary Therapies in Medicine*, 11, 156–158.

Adams, J., Lui, C-W., Sibbritt, D., Broom, A., Wardle, J., Homer, C., and Beck, S. (2009) 'Women's use of complementary and alternative medicine during pregnancy: a critical review of the literature', *Birth*, 36(3), 237–245.

Adams, J., Sibbritt, D., and Lui, C. W. (2011) 'The use of complementary and alternative medicine during pregnancy: a longitudinal study of Australian women', *Birth*, 38(3), 200–206.

Bastard, J. and Tiran, D. (2006) 'Aromatherapy and massage for antenatal anxiety: its effect on the fetus', *Complementary Therapies in Clinical Practice*, 12(1), 48–54.

Bennett, H. A., Einarson, A., Taddio, A., Koren, G. and Einarson, T. R. (2004) 'Prevalence of depression during pregnancy: systematic review', *Obstetrics & Gynecology*, 103(4), 698–709.

Bercaw, J., Maheshwari, B., and Sangi-Haghpeykar, H. (2010) 'The use during pregnancy of prescription, over-the-counter, and alternative medications among Hispanic women', *Birth*, 37(3), 211–218.

Bishop, J. L., Northstone, K., Green, J. R., and Thompson, E. A. (2011) 'The use of complementary and alternative medicine in pregnancy: data from the Avon Longitudinal Study of Parents and Children (ALSPAC)', *Complementary Therapies in Medicine*, 19(6), 303–310.

Borrelli, F., Capasso, R., Aviello, G., Pittler, M. H., and Izzo, A. A. (2005) 'Effectiveness and safety of ginger in the treatment of pregnancy-induced nausea and vomiting', *Obstetrics & Gynecology*, 105(4), 849–856.

Brown, W. J., Dobson, A. J., Bryson, L. and Byles, J. E. (1999) 'Women's health Australia: on the progress of the main cohort studies', *Journal of Women's Health and Gender-Based Medicine*, 8, 681–688.

Cagayan, M. S., and Oras, C. M. (2010) 'Use of complementary and alternative medicines among women with gestational trophoblastic diseases: a survey at the Philippine General Hospital', *The Journal of Reproductive Medicine*, 55(7–8), 327–332.

Carbone, E. T. and Zoellner, J. M. (2012) 'Nutrition and health literacy: a systematic review to inform nutrition research and practice', *Journal of the Academy of Nutrition and Dietetics*, 112(2), 254–265.

Cuzzolin, L. and Benoni, G. (2009) 'Safety issues of phytomedicines in pregnancy and paediatrics in herbal drugs'. In K.G. Ramawat (ed.) *Ethnomedicine to Modern Medicine*. Berlin: Springer Science and Business Media, pp. 381–396.

Food Standards Australia and New Zealand (FSANZ). (2013) Food standards code. Available at: www.foodstandards.gov.au/code/Pages/default.aspx

Forster, D. A., Denning, A., Wills, G., Bolger, M. and McCarthy, E. (2006) 'Herbal medicine use during pregnancy in a group of Australian women', *BMC Pregnancy and Childbirth*, 6, 21. doi: 10.1186/1471-2393-6-21.

Forster, D. A., Wills, G., Denning, A. and Bolger, M. (2009) 'The use of folic acid and other vitamins before and during pregnancy in a group of women in Melbourne, Australia', *Midwifery*, 25(2), 134–146.

Frawley, J., Adams, J., Sibbritt, D., Steel, A., Broom, A. and Gallois, C. (2013) 'Prevalence and determinants of complementary and alternative medicine use during pregnancy: results from a nationally representative sample of Australian pregnant women', *Australian and New Zealand Journal of Obstetrics and Gynaecology*, 53(4), 347–352.

Frawley, J., Adams, J., Steel, A., Broom, A., Gallois, C. and Sibbritt, D. (2015) 'Women's use and self-prescription of herbal medicine during pregnancy: an examination of 1,835 pregnant women', *Women's Health Issues*, 25(4), 396–402.

Furlow, M. L., Patel, D. A., Sen, A. and Liu, J. R. (2008) 'Physician and patient attitudes towards complementary and alternative medicine in obstetrics and gynecology', *BMC Complementary and Alternative Medicine*, 8(1), 35.

Gaffney, L. and Smith, C. (2004a) 'The views of pregnant women towards the use of complementary therapies and medicines', *Birth Issues*, 13, 43–50.

Gaffney, L. and Smith, C. (2004b)' Use of complementary therapies in pregnancy: the perceptions of obstetricians and midwives in South Australia', *Australian and New Zealand Journal of Obstetrics and Gynecology*, 44(1), 24–29.

Hall, H. G., Griffiths, D. L. and McKenna, L. G. (2011) 'The use of complementary and alternative medicine by pregnant women: a literature review', *Midwifery*, 27(6), 817–824.

Hall, H. R. and Jolly, K. (2014) 'Women's use of complementary and alternative medicines during pregnancy: a cross-sectional study', *Midwifery*, 30(5), 499–505.

Harrigan, J. T. (2011) 'Patient disclosure of the use of complementary and alternative medicine to their obstetrician/gynaecologist', *Journal of Obstetrics and Gynaecology*, 31(1), 59–61.

Hepner, D. L., Harnett, M. J., Segal, S., Camann, W., Bader, A. M., and Tsen, L. C. (2002) 'Herbal medicinal products during pregnancy: are they safe?', *BJOG: An International Journal of Obstetrics & Gynaecology*, 109(12), 1425–1426.

Hollyer, T., Boon, H., Georgousis, A., Smith, M., & Einarson, A. (2002) 'The use of CAM by women suffering from nausea and vomiting during pregnancy', *BMC Complementary and Alternative Medicine*, 2(1), 5.

Holst, L., Wright, D., Haavik, S. and Nordeng, H. (2009) 'The use and the user of herbal remedies during pregnancy', *Journal of Alternative and Complementary Medicine*, 15(7), 787–792. doi: 10.1089/aCIMCIM.2008.0467.

Hope-Allan, N., Adams, J., Sibbritt, D., and Tracy, S. (2004) 'The use of acupuncture in maternity care: a pilot study evaluating the acupuncture service in an Australian hospital antenatal clinic', *Complementary Therapies in Nursing and Midwifery*, 10(4), 229–232.

Imdad, A. and Bhutta, Z. A. (2012) 'Routine iron/folate supplementation during pregnancy: effect on maternal anaemia and birth outcomes', *Paediatric and Perinatal Epidemiology*, 26(s1), 168–177.

Kalder, M., Knoblauch, K., Hrgovic, I., and Münstedt, K. (2011) 'Use of complementary and alternative medicine during pregnancy and delivery', *Archives of Gynecology and Obstetrics*, 283(3), 475–482.

Kennedy, D. A., Lupattelli, A., Koren, G. and Nordeng, H. (2013) 'Herbal medicine use in pregnancy: results of a multinational study', *BMC Complementary and Alternative Medicine*, 13, 355. doi: 10.1186/1472-6882-13-355.

Lapi, F., Vannacci, A., Moschini, M., et al. (2010) 'Use, attitudes and knowledge of complementary and alternative drugs (CADs) among pregnant women: a preliminary survey in Tuscany', *Evidence-Based Complementary and Alternative Medicine*, 7(4), 477–486.

Lis-Balchin, M. (1999) 'Possible health and safety problems in the use of novel plant essential oils and extracts in aromatherapy', *Journal of the Royal Society of the Promotion of Health*, 119(4), 240–243.

Maats, F. H. and Crowther, C. A. (2002) 'Patterns of vitamin, mineral and herbal supplement use prior to and during pregnancy', *Australian and New Zealand Journal of Obstetrics and Gynaecology*, 42(5), 494–496.

McKenna, L. and McIntyre, M. (2006) 'What over-the-counter preparations are pregnant women taking? A literature review', *Journal of Advanced Nursing*, 56(6), 636–645.

McMahon, A. T., O'Shea, J., Tapsell, L. and Williams, P. (2014) 'What do the terms wellness and wellbeing mean in dietary practice? An exploratory qualitative study examining women's perceptions', *Journal of Human Nutrition and Dietetics*, 27(4), 401–410.

Mitchell, M. (2010) 'Risk, pregnancy and complementary and alternative medicine', *Complementary Therapies in Clinical Practice*, 16(2), 109–113.

Nordeng, H. and Havnen, G. C. (2004) 'Use of herbal drugs in pregnancy: a survey among 400 Norwegian women', *Pharmacoepidemiology and Drug Safety*, 13(6), 371–380. doi: 10.1002/pds.945.

O'Hara M. W. and McCabe, J. E. (2013) 'Postpartum depression: current status and future directions', *Annual Review of Clinical Psychology*, 9, 379–407.

Passmore, S. R. (2008) Natural rites: the culture of natural childbirth. In J. Nathanson and L. C. Tuley (eds) *Mother Knows Best: Talking Back to the Experts*. Ontario: Demeter Press.

Pettigrew, A. C., King, M. O. B., McGee, K., and Rudolph, C. (2004) 'Complementary therapy use by women's health clinic clients', *Alternative Therapies in Health and Medicine*, 10(6), 50.

SANOFI. (2016) Submission to the Public Consultation on the Review of Pharmacy Remuneration and Regulation Discussion Paper. Retrieved from https://health.gov.au/internet/main/publishing.nsf/Content/review-pharmacy-remuneration-regulation-submissions-cnt-7/$file/312-2016-09-23-sanofi-submission.pdf (accessed 7 November 2017).

Sibbritt, D. W., Catling, C. J., Adams, J., Shaw, A. J. and Homer, C. S. E. (2014) 'The self-prescribed use of aromatherapy oils by pregnant women', *Women and Birth*, 27(1), 41–45.

Skouteris, H., Wertheim, E. H., Rallis, S., Paxton, S. J., Kelly, L. and Milgrom, J. (2008) 'Use of complementary and alternative medicines by a sample of Australian women during pregnancy', *Australia and New Zealand Journal of Obstetrics and Gynaecology*, 48(4), 384–390.

Steel, A., Adams, J., Sibbritt, D., Broom, A., Frawley, J. and Gallois, C. (2014) 'Relationship between complementary and alternative medicine use and incidence of adverse birth outcomes: an examination of a nationally representative sample of 1,835 Australian women', *Midwifery*. http://dx.doi.org/10.1016/j.midw.2014.03.015.

Steel, A., Adams, J., Sibbritt, D., Broom, A., Gallois, C. and Frawley, J. (2012) 'Utilisation of complementary and alternative medicine (CAM) practitioners within maternity care provision: results from a nationally representative cohort study of 1,835 pregnant women', *BMC Pregnancy and Childbirth*, 12(1), 146.

Strouss, L., Mackley, A., Guillen, U., Paul, D. A., and Locke, R. (2014) 'Complementary and alternative medicine use in women during pregnancy: do their healthcare providers know?', *BMC Complementary and Alternative Medicine*, 14(1), 85.

TGA (Therapeutic Goods Administration). (2014) Australian regulatory guidelines for complementary medicines (ARGCIMCIM), Version 5.1.

TGA (Therapeutic Goods Administration). (2016) Australian regulation of over-the-counter medicines. Retrieved from www.tga.gov.au/australian-regulation-over-counter-medicines (accessed 7 November 2017).

Verreault, N., Da Costa, D., and Marchand, A. (2014) 'Rates and risk factors associated with depressive symptoms during pregnancy and with postpartum onset', *Journal of Psychosomatic Obstetrics & Gynecology*, 35(3), 84–91.

Wallingford, J. B., Niswander, L. A., Shaw, G. M. and Finnell, R. H. (2013) 'The continuing challenge of understanding, preventing, and treating neural tube defects', *Science*, 339(6123), 1222002.

Wardle, J. and Seely, D. (2007) The challenges of traditional, complementary and integrative medicine research: a practitioner perspective. In J. Adams (ed.) *Traditional, Complementary and Integrative Medicine: An International Reader*. New York: Palgrave Macmillan, pp. 266–282.

Warriner, S., Bryan, K. and Brown, A. M. (2014) 'Women's attitude towards the use of complementary and alternative medicines (CAM) in pregnancy', *Midwifery*, 30, 138–143.

Waterworth, S. (2011) What are flower essences? Available at: www.naturaltherapypages.com.au/article/what_are_flower_essences

Watt, G. V. D. and Janca, A. (2008) 'Aromatherapy in nursing and mental health care', *Contemporary Nurse*, 30(1), 69–75.

Westfall, R. E. (2003) 'Herbal healing in pregnancy: women's experiences', *Journal of Herbal Pharmacotherapy*, 3(4), 17–39.

# 3 Menopause and complementary and integrative medicine

## A consideration of clinical evidence, grassroots use and contemporary clinical practice guidelines

*Wenbo Peng, David Sibbritt, Amie Steel, Holger Cramer and Jon Adams*

## Introduction

Complementary and integrative medicine (CIM) use has been identified as prevalent among women for the management of menopausal symptoms, generating great interest and concern among conventional medical practitioners and health policy-makers. In this chapter, we draw upon recent quality reviews (e.g. systematic reviews with/without meta-analyses and Cochrane reviews) to investigate the empirical evidence for the efficacy of such CIM treatments as well as the prevalence, patterns, and menopausal women's decision-making of CIM use.

In addition to the clinical evidence of CIM treatments for the management of varied menopausal symptoms, this chapter also introduces contemporary guidelines on CIM use in the menopause to identify whether the 'lived' CIM use in menopause fits into the wider landscape of clinical practice guidelines for the menopause. The implications of a number of noteworthy clinical and practice-based issues are then addressed regarding CIM provision in the context of menopausal care.

## The context of the menopause

Menopause is a specific aging process of every woman referring to the permanent cessation of menstruation due to a natural decline of ovarian hormone secretion, and usually begins between the ages of 40 and 58 years with ethnic and regional variations (Shifren et al. 2014). By the year 2030, the number of menopausal women is expected to rise to 1.2 billion worldwide (Hill 1996). The common types of menopause are natural menopause and surgical menopause (World Health Organization 1996). Natural menopause refers to menopause which is not related with other pathological/physiological causes, while surgical menopause is defined as menopause induced by surgical removal of the ovaries (oophorectomy), with or without the removal of the uterus (hysterectomy). There are three stages of natural menopause. Premenopause (ambiguously used to refer to the one or two years before the menopause or the whole of the reproductive period prior to the menopause), perimenopause (the period prior to the menopause and the first year after the menopause), and postmenopause (the time dating from the final menstrual period).

Women may experience menopausal symptoms including but not limited to vasomotor symptoms (hot flushes and night sweats), mood changes (anxiety, depression, etc.), sleep problems, joint and muscle complaints, urinary disorders, and vaginal dryness (Mayo Clinic 2017). Most menopausal women experience vasomotor symptoms for seven years and many of them suffer more than ten years (Avis et al. 2015). It is worth noting that the severity of vasomotor symptoms is much higher among menopausal women aged 60–65 years compared to those of other age groups (North American Menopause Society 2015).

Menopausal symptoms generally continue after perimenopause or post-menopause and tend to have a considerable negative impact on the quality of life of both the woman and her family (Whiteley et al. 2013). Night-time awakenings following hot flushes and/or night sweats have been shown to be the main reason for work-related impairment, such as lower productivity and increased sick leave (Bolge et al. 2010). Some women experiencing severe symptomatic menopausal symptoms may leave the workforce in addition to incurring financial loss (Jack et al. 2014). Previous research has reported 40 per cent higher health-related consultation and treatment costs among women with menopausal symptoms (Fenton and Panay 2013). Such financial loss for treating menopausal symptoms also leads to a heavy economic burden on the health system (Keshishian et al. 2015).

## Conventional treatments for the menopause

Hormone therapy (HT, also known as hormone replacement therapy, HRT), oestrogen with or without progestin, is the most commonly used and most effective conventional medical treatment for the management of menopausal symptoms, in particular, vasomotor symptoms (The NAMS 2017 Hormone Therapy Position Statement Advisory Panel 2017). Prior to 2002, HT was regularly prescribed to treat menopausal symptoms (North American Menopause Society 2015). However, since the research findings of the Women's Health Initiative trial reported in 2002 the risks of HT (e.g. venous thrombo-embolism, stroke, ischaemic heart disease, and breast cancer) as outweighing therapeutical benefits, the use of HT has been debated (NAMS 2017). Also, a large proportion of women appear to avoid HT use for the management of their menopausal symptoms due to fear of potentially severe side effects (Stuenkel et al. 2012).

According to the latest North American Menopause Society (NAMS) position statement on HT use for menopause (NAMS 2017), HT is still recommended for the treatment of vasomotor symptoms and for the prevention of bone loss and fracture. To maximize the safety of HT use, HT should be considered primarily for menopausal women without contraindications to HT use and menopausal women who are within ten years of menopause or not aged over 60 years. That is, if a woman is over 60 years old or initiates HT more than ten years from menopause onset, HT becomes less favourable, owing to the greater risks of side effects (ibid.). Importantly, HT use is strongly recommended to be individualized (type, dose, duration of use) and based upon the woman's expectations as well as taking into account the personal/family medical history (Shifren et al. 2014).

## CIM in the menopause: empirical evidence for efficacy and a viable treatment alternative?

Due to the potential risks of HT for menopausal care, symptomatic menopausal women may not choose or cannot use HT doe to safety concerns. Such caution will inevitably increase the demand for alternatives that are effective and safe, and CIM therapies and products for treating menopausal symptoms have attracted research interest in recent years.

In the past five years, clinical research examining the menopause and CIM has predominantly focused upon the efficacy of acupuncture, soy products, herbal medicines, and mind-body approaches for different menopausal symptoms (Carpenter et al. 2015). Three systematic and Cochrane reviews have reported that acupuncture significantly reduces the frequency and/or severity of hot flushes when compared with no treatment. Nevertheless, there is no significant difference in efficacy on hot flushes control when comparing real and sham acupuncture (Chien et al. 2017; Chiu et al. 2016; Ee et al. 2017). Two systematic reviews have shown soy isoflavones significantly decrease the frequency and severity of hot flushes compared with placebo (Taku et al. 2012), and no significant effect on vaginal atrophy compared to various control interventions (Ghazanfarpour et al. 2016). According to a number of systematic/Cochrane reviews on black cohosh and St John's wort in menopause, black cohosh did not show significant improvements in menopausal symptoms generally compared to placebo intervention or HT (Franco et al. 2016; Laakmann et al. 2012; Leach and Moore 2008); St John's wort and its combination with black cohosh significantly reduced menopausal symptoms specifically for hot flushes in comparison to placebo (not HT) (Laakmann et al. 2012; Liu et al. 2014). Regarding mind-body approaches, no evidence was found for the alleviation of total menopausal symptoms and hot flushes exclusively with regards to the effects of hypnosis, meditation, mindfulness, tai chi or qigong, while yoga may reduce vasomotor and psychological symptoms (Goldstein et al. 2017; Shepherd-Banigan et al. 2017). Almost all the systematic reviews and the Cochrane reviews mentioned here indicate the generally low quality of relevant clinical trials, primarily owing to inadequate reporting and research design. Also, findings from such literature should be interpreted with caution, given the heterogeneity between trials.

Hot flushes are the main menopausal symptoms for which menopausal women seek CIM treatments (Kronenberg and Fugh-Berman 2002). However, the long-term safety results of CIM treatments for the management of hot flushes are largely unknown (Hickey et al. 2007), and current data are insufficient to support the efficacy of any CIM treatment for hot flushes (Nedrow et al. 2006). The CIM treatments with potential effectiveness for hot flushes suggested by individual trials warrant further study in larger rigorously-designed randomized controlled trials (RCT) to confirm the efficacy and safety of such CIM treatments and further ensure reliable comparisons between studies.

## Health services' use of CIM in the menopause

Due to a lack of solid evidence of efficacy for general or individual CIM for the management of menopausal symptoms via RCTs, many researchers have employed another rigorous research approach – health services' research (HSR) – to investigate the effectiveness and safety outcomes of CIM treatments in the field of menopausal care (Peng et al. 2014a; Peng et al. 2016). HSR refers to a range of multidisciplinary perspectives and methods, exploring the use, accessibility, cost, communication, information-seeking, and decision-making of health services for individuals, sub-groups, and populations (Adams and Steel 2012; Lohr and Steinwachs 2002). Although RCT design has been the overwhelming focus of biomedicine and CIM research to date (Staud 2011), an HSR approach is an important approach to examining all facets of the use of health care, such as the prevalence and determinants of CIM use, CIM users' profiles, and the interface between conventional medicine and CIM (Adams 2007). Along with RCT design investigation, HSR studies can help researchers fully understand the use of CIM treatments and provide a context for translating the findings of clinical trials into clinical practice (Adams et al. 2012).

Previous research has focused upon the factors regarding the rates of use and women's choices of CIM in the menopause and the motivations driving menopausal women's use of and access to CIM. As such, this section outlines the prevalence and patterns of CIM use in the menopause, as well as menopausal women's decision-making about CIM.

### *Prevalence and patterns of CIM use in the menopause*

CIM use is prevalent in menopausal care. Reviews drawing upon 2002–2012 international literature suggest that 24–91 per cent of women use CIM for menopausal symptoms (Franco et al. 2016; Peng et al. 2014a; Posadzki et al. 2013). One review also identified that 8–90 per cent of menopausal women use two or more CIM products daily (Peng et al. 2014a). Further, a study examining 30 years of menopausal women's use of CIM found the rate of CIM use approximately twice as high as the rate of HT use (Lindh-Åstrand et al. 2015). Herbal medicine, soy products and vitamins have been found to be the most frequently used CIM modalities for menopausal symptoms globally (Gartoulla et al. 2015; Ohn Mar et al. 2015; Posadzki et al. 2013).

Research shows up to half of menopausal women are frequent users of CIM without the guidance of a CIM practitioner, and concurrently use CIM and HT in menopausal care (Peng et al. 2014a; Peng et al. 2014b). A longitudinal study indicated that menopausal women were more likely to use self-prescribed CIM over time compared to CIM practitioner consultations (Peng et al. 2016). Meanwhile, concerns have been raised by conventional practitioners and researchers that self-prescribed CIM products use or concurrent use of CIM and HT may lead to adverse effects or interaction between non-hormonal managements and hormonal medications (Willis and Rayner 2013). The reasons for such concurrent use may be relevant to menopausal women's perceptions of CIM, in particular, a false perception regarding the safety of CIM remedies (Lindh-Åstrand et al. 2015).

## *Women's decision making about CIM in the menopause*

Numerous issues may account for the relative high prevalence of CIM use among menopausal women currently. Previous studies have shown menopausal women generally prefer using what they perceive to be 'natural' remedies with little or no adverse effects. CIM, especially CIM products, are often seen in this way especially when compared to HT (Australasian Menopause Society 2017; Peng et al. 2014a). In addition, many menopausal women wish to be engaged and informed with regards to their treatment options and this would appear to be a factor partly driving CIM use (Peng et al. 2014a). The perceived effectiveness of CIM modalities is another key reason for menopausal women's CIM use, with most perceiving CIM as effective in managing menopausal symptoms and further improving their quality of life (Peng et al. 2014a).

Previous literature reviews have identified consistent findings regarding the main information source of CIM used among menopausal women. To be specific, media (such as the internet, magazines, and newspapers) has been shown to be the most common source for CIM use among menopausal women (Peng et al. 2014a; Posadzki et al. 2013). In addition to media, there are a range of information sources for CIM use from the perspective of menopausal women, including friends/family members and health care practitioners (Peng et al. 2014a). However, some menopausal women perceive media-based CIM information as potentially unreliable when found via CIM product advertisements (Armitage et al. 2007). As to friends or family members constituting information sources for CIM, this refers to those women with direct or indirect positive experience in using a CIM remedy to treat their own menopausal symptoms (Williams et al. 2007).

In terms of the communication between health care practitioners and menopausal women, although practitioners are one type of information source of women's CIM use, the majority of menopausal women remain underwhelmed regarding their knowledge of CIM (Ma et al. 2006). Conventional medical practitioners' lack of CIM knowledge, hesitation to enquire about CIM use, and/or negative attitude towards CIM, are all attributed to women's self-perception as ill-informed regarding CIM use for menopausal symptoms (Stute et al. 2016). This poor communication situation can also result in a lack of disclosure of CIM use by menopausal women to their conventional medical practitioners. Research has shown 7–81 per cent of menopausal women who use CIM do not inform their health care providers about such use (Peng et al. 2014a; Posadzki et al. 2013). Furthermore, such practitioner-patient communication challenges can lead to underuse of effective CIM treatments or the use of inappropriate CIM treatments for menopausal symptoms. Thus, there seems to be a need for guidelines to facilitate conventional medical providers to effectively and safely inform their patients regarding CIM for menopausal symptoms.

## Guidelines on CIM in the menopause

As to conventional medical practitioners, the safety issue of HT and the unidentified effect of CIM options significantly complicate the situation when treating women suffering from menopausal symptoms. For this reason, clinical guidelines on CIM in menopause play an important role in highlighting best practice (De Villiers et al. 2013). While a variety of clinical trials and HSR studies on CIM for menopausal symptoms have been conducted to date, there remains only two menopause guidelines exclusively addressing CIM management of vasomotor symptoms (Carpenter et al. 2015; Mintziori et al. 2015) and two wider menopause guidelines which mention but are not exclusively focused upon CIM use (Baber et al. 2016; Cobin and Goodman 2017). These guidelines on CIM in menopause have the potential to inform conventional medical practitioners regarding the current evidence of the broad range of CIM treatment options available to menopausal women and to guide evidence-based use of CIM management of menopausal symptoms.

The exclusive menopause guidelines for CIM use are the position statements entitled *Nonhormonal Management of Menopause: Associated Vasomotor Symptoms*, released by the North American Menopause Society in 2015 (Carpenter et al. 2015) and the *EMAS Position Statement: Non-hormonal Management of Menopausal Vasomotor Symptoms*, produced by the European Menopause and Andropause Society in 2015 (Mintziori et al. 2015), respectively. The former guidelines recommend cognitive-behavioural therapy and Paroxetine salt for vasomotor symptoms, mindfulness-based stress reduction and soy products for vasomotor symptoms with caution and does not recommend yoga, vitamin supplements, herbal medicines, acupuncture, chiropractic and other CIM for vasomotor symptoms due to insufficient and inconclusive research evidence of their effects. The latter guideline supports these recommendations.

The two wider menopause guidelines, including information on CIM use, are the position statements of the International Menopause Society in 2016 (Baber et al. 2016) and the American Association of Clinical Endocrinologists and American College of Endocrinology in 2017 (Cobin and Goodman 2017), respectively. The former guidelines state that high-quality findings from studies of CIM treatments (e.g. herbal medicines, acupuncture, meditation, and cognitive behavioral therapy) for menopausal symptoms are limited, and systematic reviews and meta-analyses show inconsistent and variable efficacy results. As such, no practice recommendations are provided for CIM. In contrast, the latter guidelines report that the wider non-hormonal therapies are supported and recommended for the management of menopausal symptoms but provide no further details (Cobin and Goodman 2017).

As we know from across a number of health care fields, the success of guidelines to directly influence practice behaviour is itself not beyond controversy (Guallar and Laine 2014). Surprisingly, many CIM approaches, which are commonly used and always assumed helpful by women in the management of their menopausal symptoms as identified from empirical enquiry, do not attract recommendations in the guidelines. This context highlights the gap between CIM use and research evidence of efficacy for CIM in menopausal care, and indicates the need for further clinical research to help supplement other disciplinary approaches and establish an evidence base for CIM for menopausal symptoms. Nevertheless, the guidelines on CIM for hot flushes and night sweats currently offer some insights to help guide conventional medical practitioners with regards to selected CIM in their wider endeavours to provide menopausal women in their care with better-informed decisions on CIM.

## Future directions for CIM and the menopause

CIM use in contemporary menopausal care highlights a number of challenges for a range of stakeholders providing and receiving such care and, as identified above, the topic has attracted an emerging body of clinical and broader health services research. This section outlines a range of selected issues that require future research attention on this broad topic. While the issues outlined are not exhaustive or comprehensive, they have been chosen with a consideration for providing insights to other researchers, health care practitioners, and menopausal women themselves.

As the inconsistency regarding the use of CIM in treating menopausal symptoms between real-world CIM use (including related research output) and the menopause guidelines recommendations on different types of CIM treatments highlights, there is much to be explored from employing critical rigorous research approaches that move beyond categorizing CIM as a homogeneous group of treatments for menopausal symptoms (Adams and Robinson 2013). Indeed, the individualized nature of menopausal status, the variety of menopausal symptoms, and the broad range of heterogeneous CIM modalities make the evaluation of the effect of CIM treatments challenging via either clinical trials or HSR studies. Previous research has also suggested that CIM products and practices are far from homogeneous regarding users' ethnicity, decision-making, and needs (Kronenberg et al. 2006; Sirois and Gick 2002). Specifically, classifying menopausal women by their CIM modality type, provider type, and/or referral type may provide more insightful results in examining the use of CIM in menopause (Shmueli and Shuval 2006).

Menopausal women's self-perceived effectiveness of practitioner-administered CIM therapies and self-prescribed CIM products may account for the highly prevalent use of specific CIM treatments although they are not recommended via practitioner guidelines (Gollschewski et al. 2008). Highlighting this topic may reinforce the need for health care providers and health policy-makers to be aware of women's positive attitude towards CIM use for managing menopausal symptoms, despite a lack of robust clinical evidence from RCTs. However, the reasons for such self-perceived effectiveness of CIM is unknown. Further research is required to clarify why menopausal women choose specific CIM modalities for a certain symptom. More importantly, future in-depth research should fully examine and help understand the CIM decision-making process, treatment-seeking, and experience stratified by different menopausal symptoms.

The nature and context of communication between conventional medical practitioners and CIM practitioners constitute another area worth examining with regards to menopausal care. Some conventional medical practitioners are uncertain about the evidence of CIM therapies and products and some are reluctant to discuss CIM use with their patients, as there is scarce rigorous or high quality study findings to help them understand the efficacy of CIM modalities in menopause (Peng et al. 2014a). However, conventional medical practitioners should be aware that their negative attitudes to CIM might lead menopausal women not to disclose their CIM use, leading to possible challenges regarding direct and indirect risks (Gollschewski et al. 2008).

Given the substantial prevalence rate of self-prescribed CIM products, undoubtedly this area demands further empirical, multi-disciplinary examination, in particular with regards to the safety and possible risks of CIM product use. Although early work has begun to examine the reasons for self-prescription of CIM use among menopausal women more generally (ibid.), the exact details of self-prescribed CIM use remain unknown. In-depth investigation is needed to understand the interface between a range of medical professionals and menopausal women with regards to the safety of CIM self-prescription. Such further investigation on CIM self-prescription may also provide an opportunity for conventional medical practitioner to identify potential risks of self-prescribed CIM by menopausal women (with or without prescribed medications including HT) and to play an active role in guiding menopausal women to use appropriate CIM treatments where possible.

## Conclusion

The use of CIM is prevalent among menopausal women and the future of CIM use in treating menopausal symptoms shows some promise. To advance this important area of menopausal care, further research is needed to examine women's CIM treatment-seeking, decision-making and experience for different individual menopausal symptoms. Conventional medical providers should strive to incorporate routine clinical enquiry of CIM use when informing treatment planning for their menopausal patients.

## References

Adams, J. (2007) *Researching Complementary and Alternative Medicine*, London: Routledge.

Adams, J., Andrews, G., Barnes, J., Broom, A., and Magin, P. (2012) *Traditional, Complementary and Integrative Medicine: An International Reader*, Basingstoke: Palgrave Macmillan.

Adams, J. and Robinson, N. (2013) 'Public health and health services research in integrative medicine: an emerging, essential focus', *European Journal of Integrative Medicine*, 5(1): 1–3.

Adams, J. and Steel, A. (2012) 'Investigating complementary and alternative medicine in maternity care: The need for further public health/health services research', *Complementary Therapies in Clinical Practice*, 18(2): 73–4.

Armitage, G., Suter, E., Verhoef, M., Bockmuehl, C., and Bobey, M. (2007) 'Women's needs for CAM information to manage menopausal symptoms', *Climacteric*, 10(3): 215–24.

Australasian Menopause Society (2017) 'Complementary and herbal therapies for hot flushes'. Available at: www.menopause.org.au/hp/information-sheets/734-sleep-disturbance-and-the-menopause (accessed 5 January 2017).

Avis, N., Crawford, S., Greendale, G., et al. (2015) 'Duration of menopausal vasomotor symptoms over the menopause transition', *JAMA Internal Medicine*, 175(4): 531–9.

Baber, R., Panay, N., and Fenton, A. (2016) '2016 IMS Recommendations on women's midlife health and menopause hormone therapy', *Climacteric*, 19(2): 109–50.

Bolge, S., Balkrishnan, R., Kannan, H., Seal, B., and Drake, C. (2010) 'Burden associated with chronic sleep maintenance insomnia characterized by nighttime awakenings among women with menopausal symptoms', *Menopause*, 17(1): 80–6.

Carpenter, J., Gass, M. L., Maki, P. M., et al. (2015) 'Nonhormonal management of menopause-associated vasomotor symptoms: 2015 position statement of The North American Menopause Society', *Menopause*, 22(11): 1155–74.

Chien, T., Hsu, C., Liu, C., and Fang, C. (2017) 'Effect of acupuncture on hot flush and menopause symptoms in breast cancer: a systematic review and meta-analysis', *PloS One*, 12(8): e0180918.

Chiu, H., Shyu, Y., Chang, P., and Tsai, P. (2016) 'Effects of acupuncture on menopause-related symptoms in breast cancer survivors: a meta-analysis of randomized controlled trials', *Cancer Nursing*, 39(3): 228–37.

Cobin, R. H. and Goodman, N. F. (2017) 'American Association of Clinical Endocrinologists and American College of Endocrinology position statement on menopause – 2017 update', *Endocrine Practice*, 23: 869–80.

De Villiers, T., Pines, A., Panay, N., et al. (2013) 'Updated 2013 International Menopause Society recommendations on menopausal hormone therapy and preventive strategies for midlife health', *Climacteric*, 16(3): 316–37.

Ee, C., French, S. D., Xue, C. C., Pirotta, M., and Teede, H. (2017) 'Acupuncture for menopausal hot flashes: clinical evidence update and its relevance to decision making', *Menopause*, 24(8): 980–7.

Fenton, A. and Panay, N. (2013) 'Menopause: quantifying the cost of symptoms', *Climacteric*, 16(4): 405–6.

Franco, O. H., Chowdhury, R., Troup, J. et al. (2016) 'Use of plant-based therapies and menopausal symptoms: a systematic review and meta-analysis', *JAMA*, 315(23): 2554–63.

Gartoulla, P., Davis, S. R., Worsley, R., and Bell, R. J. (2015) 'Use of complementary and alternative medicines for menopausal symptoms in Australian women aged 40–65 years', *The Medical Journal of Australia*, 203(3): 146.

Ghazanfarpour, M., Sadeghi, R., and Roudsari, R. L. (2016) 'The application of soy isoflavones for subjective symptoms and objective signs of vaginal atrophy in menopause: a systematic review of randomised controlled trials', *Journal of Obstetrics and Gynaecology*, 36(2): 160–71.

Goldstein, K., Shepherd-Banigan, M., Coeytaux, R., et al. (2017) 'Use of mindfulness, meditation and relaxation to treat vasomotor symptoms', *Climacteric*, 20(2): 178–82.

Gollschewski, S., Kitto, S., Anderson, D., and Lyons-Wall, P. (2008) 'Women's perceptions and beliefs about the use of complementary and alternative medicines during menopause', *Complementary Therapies in Medicine*, 16(3): 163–8.

Guallar, E. and Laine, C. (2014) 'Controversy over clinical guidelines: listen to the evidence, not the noise', *Annals of Internal Medicine*, 160(5): 361–2.

Hickey, M., Saunders, C., and Stuckey, B. (2007) 'Non-hormonal treatments for menopausal symptoms', *Maturitas*, 57(1): 85–9.

Hill, K. (1996) 'The demography of menopause', *Maturitas*, 23(2): 113–27.

Jack, G., Bariola, E., Riach, K., Schnapper, J., and Pitts, M. (2014) 'Work, women and the menopause: an Australian exploratory study', *Climacteric*, 17(Suppl 2): 34.

Keshishian, A., Wang, Y., Xie, L., Baser, O., and Yuce, H. (2015) 'Examining the economic burden and health care utilization of menopausal women in the US medicaid population', *Value in Health*, 18(7): A736.

Kronenberg, F., Cushman, L., Wade, C., Kalmuss, D., and Chao, M. (2006) 'Race/ethnicity and women's use of complementary and alternative medicine in the United States: results of a national survey', *American Journal of Public Health*, 96(7): 1236–42.

Kronenberg, F. and Fugh-Berman, A. (2002) 'Complementary and alternative medicine for menopausal symptoms: a review of randomized, controlled trials', *Annals of Internal Medicine*, 137(10): 805–13.

Laakmann, E., Grajecki, D., Doege, K., zu Eulenburg, C., and Buhling, K. J. (2012) 'Efficacy of Cimicifuga racemosa, Hypericum perforatum and Agnus castus in the treatment of climacteric complaints: a systematic review', *Gynecological Endocrinology*, 28(9): 703–9.

Leach, M. J. and Moore, V. (2008) 'Black cohosh (Cimicifuga spp.) for menopausal symptoms', doi:10.1002/14651858.CD007244.pub2.

Lindh-Åstrand, L., Hoffmann, M., Hammar, M., and Spetz Holm, A. (2015) 'Hot flushes, hormone therapy and alternative treatments: 30 years of experience from Sweden', *Climacteric*, 18(1): 53–62.

Liu, Y., Jiang, Y., Huang, R., et al. (2014) 'Hypericum perforatum L. preparations for menopause: a meta-analysis of efficacy and safety', *Climacteric*, 17(4): 325–35.

Lohr, K. and Steinwachs, D. (2002) 'Health services research: an evolving definition of the field', *Health Services Research*, 37(1): 15.

Ma, J., Drieling, R., and Stafford, R. S. (2006) 'US women desire greater professional guidance on hormone and alternative therapies for menopause symptom management', *Menopause*, 13(3): 506–16.

Mayo Clinic (2017) 'Menopause'. Available at: www.mayoclinic.org/diseases-conditions/menopause/symptoms-causes/syc-20353397 (accessed 7 August 2017).

Mintziori, G., Lambrinoudaki, I., Goulis, D. G., et al. (2015) 'EMAS position statement: non-hormonal management of menopausal vasomotor symptoms', *Maturitas*, 81(3): 410–13.

Nedrow, A., Miller, J., Walker, M., et al. (2006) 'Complementary and alternative therapies for the management of menopause-related symptoms: a systematic evidence review', *Archives of Internal Medicine*, 166(14): 1453–65.

North American Menopause Society. (2015) 'The North American Menopause Society statement on continuing use of systemic hormone therapy after age 65', *Menopause*, 22(7): 693.

Ohn Mar, S., Malhi, F., Syed Rahim, S. H., Chua, C. T., Sidhu, S. S. and Sandheep, S. (2015) 'Use of alternative medications for menopause-related symptoms in three major ethnic groups of Ipoh, Perak, Malaysia', *Asia Pacific Journal of Public Health*, 27(Suppl. 8): S19–S25.

Peng, W., Adams, J., Hickman, L., and Sibbritt, D. W. (2014a) 'Complementary/alternative and conventional medicine use amongst menopausal women: Results from the Australian Longitudinal Study on Women's Health', *Maturitas*, 79(3): 340–2.

Peng, W., Adams, J., Hickman, L., and Sibbritt, D. W. (2016) 'Longitudinal analysis of associations between women's consultations with complementary and alternative medicine practitioners/use of self-prescribed complementary and alternative medicine and menopause-related symptoms, 2007–2010', *Menopause*, 23(1): 74–80.

Peng, W., Adams, J., Sibbritt, D. W., and Frawley, J. E. (2014b) 'Critical review of complementary and alternative medicine use in menopause: focus on prevalence, motivation, decision-making, and communication', *Menopause*, 21(5): 536–48.

Posadzki, P., Lee, M., Moon, T., Choi, T., Park, T., and Ernst, E. (2013) 'Prevalence of complementary and alternative medicine (CAM) use by menopausal women: a systematic review of surveys', *Maturitas*, 75(1): 34–43.

Shepherd-Banigan, M., Goldstein, K. M., Coeytaux, R. R., et al. (2017) 'Improving vasomotor symptoms; psychological symptoms; and health-related quality of life in peri- or post-menopausal women through yoga: an umbrella systematic review and meta-analysis', *Complementary Therapies in Medicine*, 34: 156–64.

Shifren, J. L., Gass, M. L. and NAMS Recommendations for Clinical Care of Midlife Women Working Group (2014) 'The North American Menopause Society recommendations for clinical care of midlife women', *Menopause*, 21(10): 1038–62.

Shmueli, A. and Shuval, J. (2006) 'Complementary and alternative medicine: Beyond users and nonusers', *Complementary Therapies in Medicine*, 14(4): 261–7.

Sirois, F. M. and Gick, M. L. (2002) 'An investigation of the health beliefs and motivations of complementary medicine clients', *Social Science & Medicine*, 55(6): 1025–37.

Staud, R. (2011) 'Effectiveness of CAM therapy: understanding the evidence', *Rheumatic Disease Clinics of North America*, 37(1): 9–17.

Stuenkel, C. A., Gass, M. L., Manson, J. E., et al. (2012) 'A decade after the Women's Health Initiative—the experts do agree', *The Journal of Clinical Endocrinology & Metabolism*, 97(8): 2617–18.

Stute, P., Ceausu, I., Depypere, H., et al. (2016) 'A model of care for healthy menopause and ageing: EMAS position statement', *Maturitas*, 92: 1–6.

Taku, K., Melby, M. K., Kronenberg, F., Kurzer, M. S. and Messina, M. (2012) 'Extracted or synthesized soybean isoflavones reduce menopausal hot flash frequency and severity: systematic review and meta-analysis of randomized controlled trials', *Menopause*, 19(7): 776–90.

The NAMS 2017 Hormone Therapy Position Statement Advisory Panel. (2017) 'The 2017 hormone therapy position statement of the North American Menopause Society', *Menopause*, 24(7): 728–53.

Whiteley, J., DiBonaventura, M., Wagner, J.-S., Alvir, J. and Shah, S. (2013) 'The impact of menopausal symptoms on quality of life, productivity, and economic outcomes', *Journal of Women's Health*, 22(11): 983–90.

Williams, R. E., Kalilani, L., DiBenedetti, D. B. et al. (2007) 'Healthcare seeking and treatment for menopausal symptoms in the United States', *Maturitas*, 58(4): 348–58.

Willis, K. F. and Rayner, J.-A. (2013) 'Integrative medical doctors: public health practitioner or lifestyle coach?', *European Journal of Integrative Medicine*, 5(1): 8–14.

World Health Organization (1996) 'Research on the menopause in the 1990s: report of a WHO scientific group'. Available at: www.who.int/iris/handle/10665/41841 (accessed 5 February, 2017).

# 4 Women, ageing and complementary and integrative medicine

*Joanna Harnett, Catherine Rickwood and Holger Cramer*

## Introduction

The aim of this chapter is to present three diverse but inextricably interwoven perspectives – sociological, pharmacological and psychophysical – for interpreting women's circumstances and behaviours as they age. Each perspective is presented within an international context and in relation to the role of complementary and integrative medicine (CIM).

According to the Global Agenda Council on Ageing Society, the 60-plus age segment is expected to increase from 11 per cent (760 million people) in 2011 to reach 22 per cent (2 billion people) by 2050 (Beard, 2011). The global population is projected to increase 3.7 times from 1950 to 2050. However, the number of individuals older than 60 and 80 years of age will increase by factors 10 and 26 respectively (ibid.). Between 2010 and 2050, the total population will increase by 2 billion, while the older population will increase by 1.3 billion creating challenges for health care users, providers and policy-makers. These challenges raise important considerations related to caring for the health of the informal caregivers in our communities.

## Women: the informal caregivers in our community: a psychosocial perspective

> It is not how much you do, but how much love you put in the doing.
>
> (Mother Theresa)

### The current situation

Informal caregiving refers to individuals who provide unpaid care to people who need assistance with activities of daily living, such as personal care, practical household help, or paperwork and/or medical tasks provided to someone living either inside or outside the carer's household (O'Reilly et al., 2008; Rodrigues et al., 2012).

Globally, the responsibility for provision of informal care (the unexpected career) to older people is primarily borne by people over 50 (Orel et al., 2007; Rodrigues et al., 2012) and it is suggested 'gender role socialization creates expectations that women in families will assume responsibility for elder as well as child caregiving' (Berg and Fugate Woods, 2009).

In Australia, more than two-thirds of those people providing informal care are female (ABS, 2016). This ratio is reflected throughout Europe, the Russian Federation and Georgia, where women over 50 years old provide between approximately 65–80 per cent of informal care of more than 20 hours per week (Rodrigues et al., 2012). In the US, it is estimated that 66 per cent of caregivers are female, with an average age of 49 (Family Caregiver Alliance, 2009). It is reasonable to assume the economic contribution of informal care by women is significant, although estimates of the value are scarce. In Australia, in 2015, the cost of replacing informal care with formal paid care was estimated at $60.3 billion, based on informal carers providing approximately 1.9 billion hours of care in 2015 (Deloitte Access Economics, 2015). Applying the ratio of informal care provision by females in Australia, the global value of care by women would be approximately $40.2 billion. The cost of replacing informal care by unskilled and skilled paid carers in the US is estimated at $221 billion and $642 billion respectively, with the opportunity cost of informal elder-care in the US estimated at $522 billion annually (Chari et al., 2015). Elsewhere in the world, the value of care has been estimated at $25 billion in Canada, €4 billion in Ireland, and €20 billion in Sweden (International Alliance of Carer Organisations, n.d.).

The role as caregiver can be physically, emotionally, socially and financially challenging, such as having an impact on the caregiver's ability to participate in social and leisure pursuits (Berg and Fugate Woods, 2009). Caregiving also has potential implications on women's health, including increased propensity to experience cardiovascular disease, elevated blood pressure and hypertension (Lee et al., 2003b). While there are also social and economic implications associated with older women's reduced ability to participate fully in the workforce (Berg and Fugate Woods, 2009, Orel et al., 2007), the focus of this chapter is on the role of older women as the caregivers in our community and the impact this has on their overall health and well-being.

## The impacts of caring

Evidence of the relationship between social isolation and mortality has long been understood (House et al., 1988). The provision of support to friends, relatives, neighbours, or a spouse, has been shown to reduce the risk of mortality (Brown et al., 2003) and have a positive effect on happiness (Nelson, et al., 2016). In fact, Poulin et al. (2013) revealed that not helping others led to a 30 per cent increased risk of mortality if exposed to a stressful life event. The reason for this positive affect may be because the provision of care has been associated with known stress-reducing hormones and neurochemicals, including oxytocin, prolactin and endogenous opioids (Poulin et al., 2013; Rodrigues et al. 2009). Furthermore, while care provision does not always have a positive effect, the provision of care provides a sense of purpose, belonging and mattering, thereby increasing happiness and reducing depression (Taylor and Turner, 2001). Social ties, social bonds and giving to others also contribute to longer, happier lives (Lakey and Orehek, 2011; Nelson et al., 2016).

When, why and how social support is given can influence its positive affect. For example, Inagaki and Orehek (2017) suggest that giving support is beneficial when given freely and perceived to be effective. Consequently, if a caregiver has a sense of obligation, the positive affect of caregiving is potentially discounted (Adelman et al., 2014). In another small-scale study of women caring for their spouses, it was revealed that caregivers consistently put their needs aside, thus leading to a divestment of health capital (Silverman, 2013). Other issues experienced by women caregivers include expectations for support being unmet, and negative interactions with the family member for whom care is provided; negative implications for the caregivers' mental health, including clinical depression and anxiety (Lee et al., 2003b); poorer immune function than controls and slower wound healing (ibid.); possible increased risk of coronary heart disease and greater cardiovascular reactivity (ibid.); elevated blood pressure (ibid.); and, feelings of guilt (Gonyea et al., 2008; Lee et al., 2003a; Neufeld and Harrison, 2003; Orel et al., 2007; Pinquart and Sorensen, 2003; Rozario and DeRienzis, 2008; Savage and Bailey, 2004). These health outcomes associated with caregiving indicate that women, as the primary caregivers in our community, risk a range of physical, mental and emotional consequences.

The extent to which a caregiver is negatively impacted by their caregiving role is influenced by the relationship between the caregiver and the care recipient (Penning and Zheng, 2016); the care recipient's disability (Clipp and George, 1993); informal social support provided to the caregiver by friends, family, and relatives; and, socioeconomic factors such as financial resources (Savage and Bailey, 2004).

### Implications of caregiving, women and an ageing population

The reason caregiving is significant and worthy of further discussion and investigation is due to our ageing population. Globally, women live longer than men. In high-income countries, women live on average six years more than men, whereas in low-income countries, the difference between men and women is three years (World Health Organization, 2014). The role of women as caretakers and their longer lives have led to what is often called "the sandwich generation" (Den-Galim and Silim, 2013) – a term coined to encompass the role women often have of simultaneously caring for their parents and children or grandchildren.

With an increasingly ageing population what does this mean for the future if older women suffer more chronic health illnesses (United Nations Secretary-General, 1999), have fewer financial resources, and yet are simultaneously the primary caregivers? Who will care for the ageing caregivers?

In their summary on women and caregiving, Berg and Fugate Woods (2009, p. 381) suggest that:

> Until economic and social parity are achieved, women around the world will continue to experience undue burden, lost opportunities, and health care systems that take advantage of their volunteer caregiving, which likely creates overall negative health consequences.

Given this challenge, the role and contribution of health professionals to ease or reduce caregiver burden are worthy of further research and investigation and it is important to acknowledge the current contribution and consider the potential contribution of CIM practitioners to alleviating the burden of care by women within an increasingly ageing population.

## Medicine use by women as they age: a pharmacological perspective

Medicine sometimes snatches away health and sometimes it gives it.

(Ovid)

Healthcare professionals clearly occupy a significant position in caring for the caregivers in our community by providing a safe confidential place to be heard and the provision of advice that enhances a woman's well-being. This will invariably involve assisting women in making informed decisions about their use of medicine.

The use of prescription and non-prescription pharmaceutical medicines increases with age, with an estimated 76 per cent of American women 60 years of age and over using two or more prescription medications and 37 per cent using five or more prescription medications (Gu, 2010). Furthermore, an estimated 65 per cent of Americans consume dietary supplements, including herbal, vitamin, mineral and nutritional supplements concurrent to prescription and/or over the counter (OTC) medication use (Qato et al., 2016). Similar patterns of medicine use have been reported in Australia (Morgan, 2012) with women aged 50 years or over consuming between one and four medicines and a third consuming between five and nine medicines (ibid.). Of the 46 per cent of individuals consuming CIM, 87.4 per cent also used prescription and over-the-counter medicines (ibid.). The specific medicines used by women >50 years of age is similar between the US (Gu, 2010), the UK (Scholes et al., 2014) and Australia (Morgan, 2012) and includes lipid lowering, antiplatelet, anti-hypertensive, anti-depressant and anti-diabetic medicines, proton pump inhibitors, analgesics and/or non-steroidal anti-inflammatory drugs (NSAIDs), and medicines used to manage asthma or chronic obstructive pulmonary disease (COPD). Not surprisingly, lipid-lowering, anti-hypertensive non-steroidal anti-inflammatory and analgesic medication use is 30 per cent higher in women who are overweight and 50 per cent higher among women who are obese compared to normoweight women (Scholes et al., 2014).

CIM promoted for cardiovascular and joint health including marine-sourced omega-3 fatty acids, glucosamine and calcium and/or vitamin D supplements are the most commonly used CIM by women aged 50 years or over in the US and Australia ( Clarke et al., 2015, Morgan, 2012; Sibbritt et al., 2016).

## Polypharmacy

> Everything in excess is opposed to nature.
>
> (Hippocrates)

Health professionals caring for women as they age are often confronted by complex clinical cases involving chronic conditions being managed via multiple medicines. The most common conditions affecting women aged 50 years or over that are managed with medicines are cardiovascular disease, hypertension and dyslipidaemia, osteoporosis diabetes and pain associated with osteoarthritis (Morgan, 2012). Polypharmacy – usually defined as the use of multiple drugs, typically >5 prescription medications (Gnjidic et al., 2012) or more than are medically necessary (Maher et al., 2014) – has known clinical consequences among older women, including a strong association with prolonged hospital stays, increased risk of food-drug interactions and falls and adverse drug interactions (Bennett et al., 2014; Maher et al., 2014; Salazar et al., 2007). Prescribing medicines for older people with polypharmacy, is often 'uncharted physiologic territory' which demands clinicians 'expect the unexpected and think of the unthinkable' (Salazar et al., 2007).

## CIM product use

Adding to the complexity of polypharmacy is the prevalent use of CIM products by women aged 50 years or over (Braun and Cohen, 2007; Maher et al., 2014; Peng et al., 2014a; Xue et al., 2007). Disclosure of medicinal CIM use is sub-optimal due to patients failing to volunteer such information and/or doctors not enquiring (Chao et al., 2008; Ducrest et al., 2017; Le et al., 2016; Liu et al., 2009; Peng et al., 2014b; Strouss et al., 2014). Less is known about the medicines history taking of CIM practitioners or the disclosure of prescription medicine use by individuals in their care.

Age-associated physiological changes that alter pharmacodynamics and pharmacokinetics have been recognised as having the potential to increase the risk of interactions in older women (Mouly et al., 2017; Sultan et al., 2015). Conversely, clinical studies suggest concurrent use of specific CIM may provide adjunctive therapeutic benefits (Conklin, 2005) or improve treatment outcomes in patients with uncontrolled treated hypertension (Ried, 2016).

Drugs used to treat cardiovascular disease, arrhythmias, and cancer tend to have complex pharmacological profiles and narrow therapeutic index. The three main ways an interaction may occur include: pharmaco-dynamic – one substance alters the sensitivity or responsiveness of tissues to another; pharmacokinetic –

a substance alters the absorption, distribution, metabolism, or excretion of a medicine; and physiochemical interactions – when two substances come into contact that are physically or chemically incompatible.

The most frequently reviewed interactions are those associated with pharmaco-dynamic alterations caused by popular herbal medicines (Sultan et al., 2015). Inhibition and induction of various cytochrome P450 enzymes and drug transporters have been identified in both *in vitro* and human studies providing evidence to support the pharmacological basis of interactions (Stieger et al., 2017). Despite this growing body of knowledge, there remains a gap in our understanding regarding the true prevalence of drug-herb interactions in older women. This may be related to the under-reporting of medicinal CIM use, the under-reporting of adverse reactions or a lack of clinical significance for many of the theoretical interactions proposed. Nevertheless, older women are more vulnerable to pharmaco-dynamic alterations and therefore the risk of harm cannot be underestimated. To care for our caregivers in the community, further research is required in this important area including:

- a need for post-market surveillance of medicinal CIM and increased vigilance in reporting suspected drug interactions and adverse reactions;
- research investigating self-prescribed and practitioner-prescribed medicinal CIM;
- the prevalence of drug-herb interactions;
- economic studies evaluating CIM practitioners' contribution to reducing polypharmacy through the provision of dietary and lifestyle advice to older women.

## Women and ageing: a psychophysical perspective

Ageing is associated with a decline in cognitive functions which is accompanied by a decline in the related neural structures (Salthouse, 2009). This decline is rather specific – those cognitive functions that are learned through early-life informa-tion processing such as vocabulary or crystallized knowledge decline only little in higher age. However, those cognitive functions that require the processing of new information decline earlier and to a much higher extent (ibid.). This is accompanied by an overall loss of white and grey neural substance with increasing age, but more specifically with an atrophy of the prefrontal cortex and the hippo-campus – structures responsible for executive function and memory (Luders, 2014: Salthouse, 2009).

The link between ageing and cognitive and neural decline is influenced by life circumstances and personal experiences, in particular by subjective stress. Chronic perceived stress reduces memory functions (Lupien et al., 2005) and reduces the function of the hippocampus, likely associated with elevated glucocorticoid levels (Conrad, 2008). Over the long term, chronically elevated cortisol levels can compromise the hippocampus by producing dendritic retraction, which is reversible when cortisol levels are reduced to normal (Conrad, 2008: Starkman et al., 1999).

Reducing chronic stress might thus be able to slow or even reverse age-related cognitive decline by reversing non-cell death-related hippocampal atrophy (Conrad, 2008). Potentially stress-reducing practices like yoga and meditation are integrated into the daily life of millions of women throughout the world. Australian research has estimated that 35 per cent of younger women use yoga and/or meditation, and 27 per cent of mid-age Australian women use these approaches (Sibbritt et al., 2011). Approximately a third of yoga users and half of meditation users cite improving memory or concentration as a major reason for starting practice (Cramer et al., 2016a; Cramer et al., 2016b). This expectation of cognition-enhancing effects, which might slow, stall, or even reverse age-related cognitive decline has been corroborated by a growing number of research studies.

Cross-sectional study participants with long-term experience in meditation report superior results in neuropsychological tests for attention, working memory, executive functions, and general information processing compared to age-matched meditation-naïve controls (Gard et al., 2014a). In one study, mid-age meditators even outperformed younger controls regarding temporal attention (van Leeuwen et al., 2009). Using a more comprehensive approach to cognitive function, Gard et al. (2014b) tested differences between yoga and meditation practitioners and age-matched controls on fluid intelligence – cognitive functions needed to solve unknown problems, independent of any previously acquired knowledge. The study demonstrated that meditation/yoga practitioners had a less pronounced age-related decline in fluid intelligence than control. Yogis even had less decline than mediators, probably due to the known neuroprotective effects of physical activity that are combined with meditation in yoga practice. Across groups, higher values in mindfulness were associated with less age-related decline (ibid.).

Further studies have compared brain images of meditation practitioners and non-practitioners and found age-related decreases in white and grey matter in the latter group while experienced meditation practitioners show no such decrease (Lazar et al., 2005; Luders et al., 2011; Pagnoni and Cekic, 2007). One study even found hints of an *increase* of total grey matter volume with increasing age among meditation practitioners, potentially related to preservation of existing neurons but also to neuroplasticity (Pagnoni and Cekic, 2007). The authors of one of the studies concluded that 'the average cortical thickness of the 40- to 50-year old meditation participants was similar to the average thickness of the 20- to 30-year-old meditators and controls' (Lazar et al., 2005). However, meditation practice is not simply a binary issue (practice or no practice) and the frequency and content of meditation seem to be significant. Employing magnetic resonance imaging, Villemure et al. (2015) found age-related grey matter decline in the prefrontal cortex and the hippocampus only for non-yoga practitioners suggesting possible neuroprotective effects of yoga. This work also reported yoga practice (especially the combination of yoga postures and meditation) frequency as correlating with grey matter volume in the hippocampus and other brain areas (ibid.).

While these findings are intriguing, they are nevertheless limited. While meditation may well decrease age-related decline and lead to better cognitive function in older age, the explanation might also well be the other way around: since meditation requires attention and concentration, it is also possible that only people with strong cognitive function initiate and maintain meditation practice. Moreover, since research often tries to maximize differences between groups, most studies used meditators with decades of practice rendering the application of their findings to the standard casual mediator or even individuals with cognitive impairments a challenge.

In order to address these issues, several longitudinal studies allocated a number of mid- to higher-age participants to a standardized meditation intervention and others to an alternative intervention – ideally via random allocation. These studies demonstrate increases in general cognitive function, attention, memory and executive functions in the participants allocated to meditation compared to controls after only a few weeks of meditation practice ( Alexander et al., 1989; Lavretsky et al., 2013; McHugh et al., 2010, Moynihan et al., 2013, Oken et al., 2010, Sun et al., 2013) and report executive function as improving immediately following a mindfulness meditation intervention as short as 15 minutes compared to a time-matched non-meditation practice (McHugh et al., 2010). Lavretsky et al. (2013) compared the effects of the yoga-based Kirtan Kriya meditation to a relaxation condition (listening to relaxation music) in older family dementia caregivers with depressive symptoms, reporting that the meditation group had a stronger increase than the control group with regard to overall cognitive function and more specifically in executive functions. Interestingly, the meditation group also exhibited a substantially stronger increase in telomerase activity (ibid.), an enzyme that promotes cell longevity by counteracting the shortening of telomeres, a protective protein capping the ends of human chromosomes (Epel et al., 2009; Lin et al., 2009). Shortening of telomeres is thought to be indicative of bodily ageing and has been associated with a number of chronic diseases such as dementia and cardio-vascular disease (Epel et al., 2009). Such a finding can possibly be regarded as a first suggestion, albeit with much room for further evaluation, that yoga and meditation may not only slow age-related cognitive decline but perhaps even ageing itself.

Neural decline with increasing age may also be counteracted by meditation. Holzel et al. (2008) obtained anatomical magnetic resonance images from healthy mid-age meditation-naïve participants before and after undertaking an 8-week mindfulness meditation intervention identifying an increase of hippocampal grey matter when compared to a waiting list control group (ibid.).

In conclusion, meditation seems to slow, stall, and sometimes even reverse age-related cognitive decline as well as a decline in related neural structures, potentially by reducing subjective stress and increasing mindfulness. However, the usefulness of meditation as a therapy for dementia is questionable due the obvious challenges of people with dementia to successfully practise meditation, and meditation may be more suitable as a means to counter normal age-related decline with the combination of active and passive meditation (such as in yoga) seeming to be particularly effective. In this area of enquiry, further research is required to compare different forms of meditation impact on specific cognitive effects and to investigate the relationship between the time point (i.e. age of initiating meditation), time spent meditating and the prevention of cognitive decline.

## Conclusion

As women age, the physical and psychosocial demands increase. Women are playing an increasing significant part in caring for the ageing population as they face their own challenges associated with ageing themselves. Health care professionals need to be aware of these challenges and sensitive to the needs of the women for whom they care. Women's use of medicines, including CIM, plays an important role in the prevention and management of age-related disease. However, substantial use of prescription and CIM products is largely 'unchartered physiological territory' that requires judicious care and further research to reduce unwanted outcomes. Finally, the potential benefits of low-risk psychophysical practices such as yoga and meditation cannot be ignored as providing potential preventative and therapeutic benefits for women as they age.

## References

Adelman, R. D., Tmanova, L. L., Delgado, D., Dion, S. and Lachs, M. S. 2014. Caregiver burden: a clinical review. *The Journal of the American Medical Association*, 311, 1052–1060.

Alexander, C. N., Langer, E. J., Newman, R. I., Chandler, H. M. and Davies, J. L. 1989. Transcendental meditation, mindfulness, and longevity: an experimental study with the elderly. *Journal of Personality and Social Psychology*, 57, 950–964.

Australian Bureau of Statistics, 2016. *Disability, Ageing and Carers, Australia: Summary of Findings, 2015.* Catalogue No. 4430.0.

Beard, J. R. 2011. *Global Population Ageing: Peril or Promise.* Geneva: World Economic Forum.

Bennett, A., Gnjidic, D., Gillett, M., et al. 2014. Prevalence and impact of fall-risk-increasing drugs, polypharmacy, and drug–drug interactions in robust versus frail hospitalised falls patients: a prospective cohort study. *Drugs & Aging*, 31, 225–232.

Berg, J. A. and Fugate Woods, N. 2009. Global women's health: a spotlight on caregiving. *Nursing Clinics of North America*, 44, 375–384.

Braun, L. and Cohen, M. 2007. Australian hospital pharmacists' attitudes, perceptions, knowledge and practices of CAMs. *Journal of Pharmacy Practice and Research*, 37, 220–223.

Brown, S. L., Nesse, R. M., Vinokur, A. D. and Smith, D. M. 2003. Providing social support may be more beneficial than receiving it: results from a prospective study of mortality. *Psychological Science*, 14, 320–327.

Chao, M. T., Wade, C. and Kronenberg, F. 2008. Disclosure of complementary and alternative medicine to conventional medical providers: variation by race/ethnicity and type of cam. *Journal of the National Medical Association*, 100, 1341–1349.

Chari, A. V., Engberg, J., Ray, K., N. and Mehrotra, A. 2015. The opportunity costs of informal elder-care in the United States: new estimates from the American time use survey. *Health Services Research*, 50, 871–882.

Clarke, T. C., Black, L. I., Stussman, B. J., Barnes, P. M. and Nahin, R. L. 2015. Trends in the use of complementary health approaches among adults: United States, 2002–2012. *National Health Statistics Reports*, 1.

Clipp, E. and George, L. 1993. Dementia and cancer: a comparison of spouse caregivers. *Gerontologist*, 33, 534–541.

Conklin, K. A. 2005. Coenzyme Q10 for prevention of anthracycline-induced cardiotoxicity. *Integrative Cancer Therapies*, 4, 110–130.

Conrad, C. D. 2008. Chronic stress-induced hippocampal vulnerability: the glucocorticoid vulnerability hypothesis. *Review of Neuroscience*, 19, 395–411.

Cramer, H., Hall, H., Leach, M., et al. 2016a. Prevalence, patterns, and predictors of meditation use among US adults: a nationally representative survey. *Science Reports*, 6, 36760.

Cramer, H., Ward, L., Steel, A., et al. 2016b. Prevalence, patterns, and predictors of yoga use: results of a U.S. nationally representative survey. *American Journal of Preventative Medicine*, 50, 230–235.

Deloitte Access Economics 2015. The economic value of informal care in Australia in 2015.

Den-Galim, D. and Silim, A. 2013. *The Sandwich Generation: Older Women Balancing Work and Care*. London: Institute of Public Policy Research.

Ducrest, I., Marques-Vidal, P., Faouzi, M., et al. 2017. Complementary medicine use among general internal medicine inpatients in a Swiss university hospital. *International Journal of Clinical Practice*, e12952-n/a.

Epel, E., Daubenmier, J., Moskowitz, J. T., Folkman, S. and Blackburn, E. 2009. Can meditation slow rate of cellular aging? Cognitive stress, mindfulness, and telomeres. *Annals of New York Academy of Science*, 1172, 34–53.

Gard, T., Holzel, B. K. and Lazar, S. W. 2014a. The potential effects of meditation on age-related cognitive decline: a systematic review. *Annals of New York Academy of Science*, 1307, 89–103.

Gard, T., Taquet, M., Dixit, R., et al. 2014b. Fluid intelligence and brain functional organization in aging yoga and meditation practitioners. *Frontiers in Aging Neuroscience*, 6, 76.

Gnjidic, D., Hilmer, S. N., Blyth, F. M., et al. 2012. Polypharmacy cutoff and outcomes: five or more medicines were used to identify community-dwelling older men at risk of different adverse outcomes. *Journal of Clinical Epidemiology*, 65, 989–995.

Gonyea, J. G., Paris, R. and Zerden, L. D. S. 2008. Adult daughters and aging mothers: the role of guilt in the experiences of caregiver burden. *Aging and Mental Health*, 12, 559–567.

Gu Q, D. C. and Burt V. 2010. Prescription drug use continues to increase: US prescription drug data for 2007–2008. In National Center for Health Statistics (ed.). *Statistics*. Hyattsville: NCHS.

Holzel, B. K., Ott, U., Gard, T., et al. 2008. Investigation of mindfulness meditation practitioners with voxel-based morphometry. *Social Cognitive and Affective Neuroscience*, 3, 55–61.

House, J. S., Landis, K. R. and Umberson, D. 1988. Social relationships and health. *Science*, 241, 540–545.

Inagaki, T.K. and Orehek, E. 2017. On the benefits of giving social support: When, why and how support providers gain by caring for others. *Current Direction in Psychological Science*, 26(2), 109–113.

International Alliance of Carer Organisations. n.d. *Global Carer Facts* [Online]. Available at: www.internationalcarers.org/carer-facts/global-carer-stats/ (accessed 5 June, 2017).

Lakey, B. and Orehek, E. 2011. Relational regulation theory: a new approach to explain the link between perceived social support and mental health. *Psychological Review*, 118, 482–495.

Lavretsky, H., Epel, E. S., Siddarth, P., et al. 2013. A pilot study of yogic meditation for family dementia caregivers with depressive symptoms: effects on mental health, cognition, and telomerase activity. *International Journal of Geriatric Psychiatry*, 28, 57–65.

Lazar, S. W., Kerr, C. E., Wasserman, R. H., et al. 2005. Meditation experience is associated with increased cortical thickness. *Neuroreport*, 16, 1893–1897.

Le, T. Q., Smith, L. and Harnett, J. 2016. A systematic review: biologically-based complementary medicine use by people living with cancer, is a more clearly defined role for the pharmacist required? *Research in Social and Administrative Pharmacy*, 13(6), 1037–1044.

Lee, S., Colditz, G., Berkman, L. and Kawachi, I. 2003a. Caregiving to children and grandchildren and risk of coronary heart disease in women. *American Journal of Public Health*, 93, 1939–1944.

Lee, S., Colditz, G. A., Berkman, L. F. and Kawachi, I. 2003b. Caregiving and risk of coronary heart disease in U.S. women: a prospective study. *American Journal of Preventive Medicine*, 24, 113–119.

Lin, J., Epel, E. S. and Blackburn, E. H. 2009. Telomeres, telomerase stress and aging. In: Bernston, G. G. and Cacioppo, J. T. (eds.) *Handbook of Neuroscience for the Behavioral Sciences*. Hoboken, NJ: Wiley.

Liu, C., Yang, Y., Gange, S. J., et al. 2009. Disclosure of complementary and alternative medicine use to health care providers among HIV-infected women. *AIDS Patient Care and STDs*, 23, 965–971.

Luders, E. 2014. Exploring age-related brain degeneration in meditation practitioners. *Annals of the New York Academy of Science*, 1307, 82–88.

Luders, E., Clark, K., Narr, K. L. and Toga, A. W. 2011. Enhanced brain connectivity in long-term meditation practitioners. *Neuroimage*, 57, 1308–1316.

Lupien, S. J., Fiocco, A., Wan, N., et al. 2005. Stress hormones and human memory function across the lifespan. *Psychoneuroendocrinology*, 30, 225–242.

Maher, R. L., Hanlon, J. and Hajjar, E. R. 2014. Clinical consequences of polypharmacy in elderly. *Expert Opinion on Drug Safety*, 13, 57–65.

McHugh, L., Simpson, A. and Reed, P. 2010. Mindfulness as a potential intervention for stimulus over-selectivity in older adults. *Research in Developmental Disabilities*, 31, 178–184.

Morgan, T. K. 2012. A national census of medicines use: a 24-hour snapshot of Australians aged 50 years and older. *Medical Journal of Australia*, 196, 50–53.

Mouly, S., Lloret-Linares, C., Sellier, P.-O., Sene, D. and Bergmann, J.-F. 2017. Is the clinical relevance of drug-food and drug-herb interactions limited to grapefruit juice and Saint-John's Wort? *Pharmacological Research*, 118, 82–92.

Moynihan, J. A., Chapman, B. P., Klorman, R., et al. 2013. Mindfulness-based stress reduction for older adults: effects on executive function, frontal alpha asymmetry and immune function. *Neuropsychobiology*, 68, 34–43.

Nelson, S. K., Layous, K., Cole, S. W. and Lyumbomirsky, S. 2016. Do unto others or treat yourself? The effects of prosocial and self-focused behavior on psychological flourishing. *Emotion*, 16, 850–861.

Neufeld, A. and Harrison, M. J. 2003. Unfulfilled expectations and negative interactions: nonsupport in the relationships of women caregivers. *Journal of Advanced Nursing*, 41, 323–331.

Oken, B. S., Fonareva, I., Haas, M., et al. 2010. Pilot controlled trial of mindfulness meditation and education for dementia caregivers. *Journal of Alternative and Complementary Medicine*, 16, 1031–1038.

O'Reilly, D., Connolly, S., M., R. and Patterson, C. 2008. Is caring associated with an increased risk of mortality? A longitudinal study. *Social Science and Medicine*, 67, 1282–1290.

Orel, N. A., Landry-Meyer, L. and Spence, M. A. S. 2007. Women's caregiving careers and retirement financial insecurity. *Adultspan Journal*, 6, 49–62.

Pagnoni, G. and Cekic, M. 2007. Age effects on gray matter volume and attentional performance in Zen meditation. *Neurobiology of Aging*, 28, 1623–1627.

Peng, W., Adams, J., Hickman, L. and Sibbritt, D. W. 2014a. Complementary/alternative and conventional medicine use amongst menopausal women: results from the Australian Longitudinal Study on Women's Health. *Maturitas*, 79, 340–342.

Peng, W., Adams, J., Sibbritt, D. W. and Frawley, J. E. 2014b. Critical review of complementary and alternative medicine use in menopause: focus on prevalence, motivation, decision-making, and communication. *Menopause*, 21, 536–548.

Penning, M. J. and Zheng, W. 2016. Caregiver stress and mental health: impact of caregiving relationship and gender. *Gerontologist*, 56, 1102–1113.

Pinquart, M. and Sorensen, S. 2003. Differences between caregivers and noncaregivers in psychological health and physical health: a meta-analysis. *Psychology and Aging*, 18, 250–267.

Poulin, M. J., Brown, S. L., Dillard, A. J. and Smith, D. M. 2013. Giving to others and the association between stress and mortality. *American Journal of Public Health*, 103, 1649 1655.

Qato, D. M., Wilder, J., Schumm, L. P., Gillet, V. and Alexander, G. C. 2016. Changes in prescription and over-the-counter medication and dietary supplement use among older adults in the United States, 2005 vs 2011. *JAMA Internal Medicine*, 176, 473–482.

Ried, K. 2016. Garlic lowers blood pressure in hypertensive individuals, regulates serum cholesterol, and stimulates immunity: an updated meta-analysis and review. *The Journal of Nutrition*, 146, 389S–396S.

Rodrigues, R., Huber, M. and Lamura, G. E. 2012. *Facts and Figures on Healthy Ageing and Long-term Care*. Vienna: European Centre for Social Welfare Policy and Research.

Rodrigues, S. M., Saslow, L. R., Garcia, N., John, O. P. and Keltner, D. 2009. Oxytocin receptor genetic variation relates to empathy and stress reactivity in humans. *Proceedings of the National Academy of Sciences*, 106, 210437–21441.

Rozario, P. A. and DeRienzis, D. 2008. Familism beliefs and psychological distress among African American women caregivers. *Gerontologist*, 48, 772–780.

Salazar, J. A., Poon, I. and Nair, M. 2007. Clinical consequences of polypharmacy in elderly: expect the unexpected, think the unthinkable. *Expert Opinion on Drug Safety*, 6, 695–704.

Salthouse, T. A. 2009. Decomposing age correlations on neuropsychological and cognitive variables. *Journal of International Neuropsychological Society*, 15, 650–661.

Savage, S. and Bailey, S. 2004. The impact of caring on caregivers' mental health: a review of the literature. *Australian Health Review*, 27, 111–117.

Scholes, S., Faulding, S. and Mindell, J. 2014. *Use of Prescribed Medicines: NHS Health Survey for England–2013*. London: Health & Social Care Information Centre, 2.

Sibbritt, D., Adams, J. and Van Der Riet, P. 2011. The prevalence and characteristics of young and mid-age women who use yoga and meditation: results of a nationally representative survey of 19,209 Australian women. *Complementary Therapies in Medicine*, 19, 71–77.

Sibbritt, D., Lui, C., Kroll, T. and Adams, J. 2016. Prevalence of glucosamine and omega-3 fatty acid use and characteristics of users among mid-age women: analysis of a nationally representative sample of 10,638 women. *The Journal of Nutrition, Health & Aging*, 20, 637–644.

Silverman, M. 2013. Sighs, smiles, and worried glances: how the body reveals women caregivers' lived experiences of care to older adults. *Journal of Aging Studies*, 27, 288–297.

Starkman, M. N., Giordani, B., Gebarski, S. S., et al. 1999. Decrease in cortisol reverses human hippocampal atrophy following treatment of Cushing's disease. *Biological Psychiatry*, 46, 1595–1602.

Stieger, B., Mahdi, Z. M. and Jäger, W. 2017. Intestinal and hepatocellular transporters: therapeutic effects and drug interactions of herbal supplements. *Annual Review of Pharmacology and Toxicology*, 57, 399–416.

Strouss, L., Mackley, A., Guillen, U., Paul, D. A. and Locke, R. 2014. Complementary and alternative medicine use in women during pregnancy: do their healthcare providers know? *BMC Complementary and Alternative Medicine*, 14, 85.

Sultan, S., Viqar, M., Ali, R., Tajik, A. J. and Jahangir, A. 2015. Essentials of herb-drug interactions in the elderly with cardiovascular disease. *Journal of Patient-Centered Research and Reviews*, 2, 174–191.

Sun, J., Kang, J., Wang, P. and Zeng, H. 2013. Self-relaxation training can improve sleep quality and cognitive functions in the older: a one-year randomised controlled trial. *Journal of Clinical Nursing*, 22, 1270–1280.

Taylor, J. and Turner, R. 2001. A longitudinal study of the role and significance of mattering to others for depressive symptoms. *Journal of Health and Social Behaviour*, 42, 310–325.

United Nations Secretary-General. 1999. *Gender and Ageing: Problems, Perceptions and Policies* [Online]. Available at: www.un.org/womenwatch/daw/csw/aging.htm (accessed 15 June 2017).

Van Leeuwen, S., Muller, N. G. and Melloni, L. 2009. Age effects on attentional blink performance in meditation. *Consciousness and Cognition*, 18, 593–599.

Villemure, C., Ceko, M., Cotton, V. A. and Bushnell, M. C. 2015. Neuroprotective effects of yoga practice: age-, experience-, and frequency-dependent plasticity. *Frontiers of Human Neuroscience*, 9, 281.

World Health Organization. 2014. *World Health Statistics 2014* [Online]. Available at: www.who.int/meiacentre/news/releases/2014/world-health-statistics-2014/en/ (accessed 15 June, 2017).

Xue, C., Zhang, A., Lin, V., Da Costa, C. and Story, D. 2007. Complementary and alternative medicine use in Australia: a national population-based survey. *Journal of Alternative and Complementary Medicine*, 13, 643–650.

# Part II

# CIM use and women's health issues

# 5 Women's cancers and complementary and integrative medicine

## A focus upon prevention, disease management and survivorship

*Janet Schloss, Lise Alschuler and Ellen McDonell*

## Overview

The use of complementary and integrative medicine (CIM) before, during, and after cancer treatment has become increasingly common, with approximately 40 per cent of individuals with cancer using CIM (Horneber et al., 2012). Women with cancer are more likely to use CIM therapies than men (Hedderson et al. 2004), and in particular women with breast cancer are among the heaviest CIM users with use reported at over 75 per cent (Greenlee et al., 2009).

For most, a truly alternative approach to cancer is not sought by patients nor advised by clinicians; therefore, the term integrative oncology is often used. Integrative oncology (IO) is defined as a "patient-centred, evidence-informed field of cancer care that utilizes mind and body practices, natural products, and/or lifestyle modifications from different traditions alongside conventional cancer treatments". Integrative oncology aims to optimize health, quality of life, and clinical outcomes from across the cancer care continuum and to empower people to prevent cancer and become active participants before, during, and beyond cancer treatment (Witt et al., 2017).

CIM and IO encompass a wide variety of modalities; five broad categories established by the National Institute of Health's National Centre for Complementary and Alternative Medicine (NCCAM) are often referenced in the literature (Deng et al., 2009, Wai., 2005). These categories are: (1) biologically based therapies (e.g. herbal remedies, dietary supplements); (2) mind-body techniques (e.g. meditation, hypnotherapy, support groups); (3) manipulative and body-based practices (e.g. massage, exercise); (4) energy therapies (e.g. Reiki, qi gong); and (5) ancient or whole medical systems (e.g. traditional Chinese medicine (TCM), Ayurvedic medicine, naturopathic medicine). These categories are not distinct.

This chapter argues there is a need for a greater focus on CIM and women's cancers. It exemplifies that women are more likely to use CIM and access CIM practitioners to assist their treatment and future. Currently, there is limited attention on women's cancer and CIM and this chapter is a direct response to the gap in the research and knowledge. CIM can play a major role in assisting the prevention, aid as an adjunct to treatment and increase longevity of women diagnosed with cancer.

## Introduction

Cancer, malignant tumours or neoplasms are generic terms for a group of diseases which are all characterized by the growth of abnormal cells (WHO, 2017b). Cancer is the second leading cause of death globally with the most common cancers for women consisting of breast, colorectal, lung, cervix and stomach cancer (ibid.). According to the World Health Organisation (WHO), the incidence rates vary greatly worldwide for women's cancer with breast cancer, for example, varying from 19.3 per 100,000 women in Eastern Africa to 89.7 per 100,000 women in Western Europe (WHO, 2017a). It is estimated that the number of new cases of cancer is expected to rise by about 70 per cent over the next two decades (WHO, 2017b).

Among the cancer cases diagnosed, approximately one-third of the deaths from cancer are due to the five leading behavioural and dietary risks: high body mass index; low fruit and vegetable intake; lack of physical activity; tobacco consumption; and alcohol consumption (ibid.). The WHO estimate that 30–50 per cent of cancers could be prevented if these lifestyle and behavioural risk factors were addressed (ibid.). The four leading women's cancers – breast, colorectal, lung and gynaecological – all involve lifestyle and behavioural risk factors that CIM can assist.

## Cancer prevention strategies incorporating CIM

The majority of research on cancer is focused on treatment and prevention of recurrence. For the prevention of the development of cancer, the research is based on reducing risk factors. The main CIM strategies incorporated into cancer prevention include diet, exercise and environmental mitigation which will be expanded on below.

### *Diet*

There are several dietary patterns and specific nutrients associated with a reduction of cancer risk. One of the main components of CIM is dietary changes and focusing on diet has the capacity to prevent cancer in women. Examining the broader body of research on CIM dietary changes and cancer, a common denominator is a plant-based diet (Shapira, 2017). Fruit, vegetables, and certain components of plant foods, such as fibre and polyphenols, have a large body of data supporting a protective effect against cancer (Bradbury, 2014). Adherence to a Mediterranean diet (a diet high in plant foods, as well as olive oil, fish, and moderate wine) has been found to be associated with reduced risk of cancer incidence (Benetou et al., 2008). The impact of this general dietary pattern of a plant-based diet has also been studied in specific cancer patient populations (Romagnolo and Selmin, 2017).

Specific to women, changes in dietary patterns to either decrease energy from fat or to increase fibre intake can alter the enterohepatic recirculation of oestrogens, leading to lower circulating oestrogen concentrations, in turn, lending a protective effect against oestrogen receptor positive tumours (Narita et al., 2017). A low-fat/high-fibre diet can reduce serum oestradiol by an average of 7.5 per cent (Gann et al., 2003), an effect of particular importance to women with a prior history of oestrogen receptor positive breast cancer. The polyphenolics found in plant-based diets such as quercetin, genistein, curcumin, and resveratrol are also of importance to women as they have been found to reduce the risk of certain cancers (Sun et al., 2017). Soy isoflavones in particular have been found to be beneficial for breast cancer reduction although soy has also been quite controversial (Kwon, 2014). A pooled analysis of three large prospective trials assessed the impact of soy isoflavones by country on the risk of recurrence (Nechuta et al., 2012). This large research project showed a consumption of ≥10 mg isoflavones per day was associated with a 25 per cent reduced risk of recurrence of breast cancer, particularly for those of Asian background (ibid.).

Ovarian cancer risk has been found to be affected by diet (Wang et al., 2017). A systematic meta-analysis assessing the relationship between dietary patterns and the risk of ovarian cancer (ibid.) found evidence of a decreased risk for ovarian cancer following a healthy dietary pattern[1] and an increased risk of ovarian cancer for those following a western-style diet.[2] Similarly, frequent consumption of red meat, refined carbohydrates, dairy and eggs is associated with an increased risk of developing colorectal cancer compared to infrequent consumption (Bidoli et al., 1992). There is also a significant inverse relationship between total fibre intake and risk of colorectal cancer. Vegetable fibre appears to be more protective than either fruit or grain fibre (Levi et al., 2001). Obesity is a known risk factor for colorectal cancer. Obesity-related dyslipidemias, increased adipokines and elevated insulin and insulin-like growth factor-1 are collectively associated with both increased colorectal cancer incidence and mortality in both men and women (Muc-Wierzgoń et al., 2014). Lastly, an inflammatory diet which consists of a high consumption of red and processed meats, high consumption of refined and processed foods, low consumption in fruit and vegetables, nuts and seeds, healthy oils and fish has been found to increase the risk of colorectal cancer in a meta-analysis (Fan et al., 2017).

## *Physical activity*

Exercise is a critical component of a lifestyle-based CIM support cancer prevention programme. Women who engaged in the equivalent of at least two to three hours of brisk walking each week in the year before they were diagnosed with breast cancer were 31 per cent less likely to die of the disease than women who were sedentary before their diagnosis (Irwin et al., 2008). A prospective cohort study also identified that, for individuals with colon cancer, engaging in 8.75 or more hours per week in recreational physical activity (equivalent to 150 mins/week of walking) compared to 3.5 hours per week was associated with lower all-cause mortality, whereas sitting 6 or more hours per day during leisure time compared to less than 3 hours per day was associated with a higher all-cause mortality (Campbell et al., 2013). A meta-analysis examining 5-year mortality for women with ovarian cancer has found inactive women (women with no regular weekly recreational physical activity) with residual disease were at a 34 per cent increased risk of mortality and inactive women without residual disease had a 22 per cent increased risk of mortality (Cannioto et al., 2016). These studies serve as a reminder that the impact of physical activity on cancer risk encompasses a continuum inclusive of a sedentary lifestyle and regular exercise.

## *Environment*

There are several environmental factors that can present serious risk to human health with a growing body of evidence linking exposure to certain environmental and occupational pollutants to cancer (Perduca et al., 2018). Some of these environmental and occupational pollutants may be able to be mitigated by CIM practices such as dietary choices (Muscaritoli et al., 2016) and biologics.

A significant pathway from environmental toxins to carcinogenesis is through endocrine disruption. According to the National Institute of Environmental Health Sciences (NIEHS), chemicals that are confirmed endocrine disruptors in humans include diethylstilbestrol (DES), dioxin and dioxin-like compounds, polychlorinated biphenyls (PCBs), DDT and other pesticides, bisphenol A (BPA), and di(2-ethylhexyl) phthalate (DEHP). Phthalates, which are industrial chemicals found in nearly any product that has synthetic fragrance, are also known endocrine disruptors (NIEHS, 2010).

Chemicals that disrupt hormone function have the ability to modify hormonal signalling throughout the body and impact the progression of cancer (ibid.). Thus, avoiding exposure to these types of environmental carcinogens will decrease the risk of cancers connected with these toxins. In addition, CIM may be able to assist in the detoxification of these hormone-disrupting chemicals such as the use of 3,3'-diindolylmethane (DIM) which has been found to be capable of detoxifying carcinogens linked to breast cancer (Chen et al., 2016).

## Cancer management strategies and CIM

During cancer treatment, CIM are commonly used with the goals of improving wellness, enhancing quality of life, and relieving symptoms of disease and the side effects of conventional treatments (Greenlee et al., 2017). While there are many potentially useful therapies with varying degrees of evidence, the following is a sample of some of the more evidence-based CIM that may be suitable for women with cancer.

Mind-body therapies are beneficial for a variety of symptoms including anxiety, depression, insomnia, and quality of life (Carlson et al., 2017). In particular, meditation and mindfulness based therapies (Haller et al., 2017), cognitive-behavioural therapy (CBT) (Xiao et al., 2017), and yoga therapy (Cramer et al., 2017) have good evidence supporting their use in cancer. Mind-body approaches are not only beneficial for emotional wellness outcomes, but evidence suggests they may also impact survival outcomes (Stagl et al., 2015). One mechanism through which mind-body therapies exert their effect is through changes in physiological markers of stress and inflammation including cortisol, C-reactive protein, and tumour necrosis factor alpha (Lopresti, 2017), indicating improvements in sympathetic nervous system and hypothalamic-pituitary axis functioning (Pascoe et al., 2017).

Body-based therapies such as massage therapy and exercise have research-based utility in cancer management. Research on massage therapy has shown moderate impact on anxiety and depressive symptoms (Krohn et al., 2011), although a Cochrane review found the quality of evidence to be poor and thus conclusions could not be drawn regarding the impact for pain, anxiety, depression and stress (Shin et al., 2016). Appropriate exercise should be recommended for all individuals with cancer to support quality of life, and aerobic and muscular fitness (Segal et al., 2017).

Acupuncture, a component of traditional Chinese medicine, has been studied and used clinically for management of cancer symptoms and its side effects. Currently, the best evidence for acupuncture and acupressure is for cancer-related fatigue (Zhang et al., 2017), aromatase-inhibitor-induced arthralgia (Chen et al., 2017), and chemotherapy-induced nausea and vomiting (CINV) (Dibble et al., 2007; Molassiotis et al., 2007). In women with gynaecological cancer being treated with chemotherapy, acupuncture to PC6 prior to chemotherapy compared to ondansetron 8 mg, resulted in significantly reduced delayed-onset nausea, fewer additional doses of ondansetron, and fewer adverse effects including constipation and insomnia (Rithirangsriroj et al., 2015). Acupuncture and acupressure may also be beneficial in reducing post-operative nausea and vomiting (PONV), although more research is warranted (Lee, 2015).

Evidence for the use of biologically-based treatments has generally been weaker and less robust. However, there are many therapies with promising and emerging evidence for use during cancer treatment. In women with breast cancer, *Panax quinquefolius* (American ginseng) has been found to significantly reduce cancer-related fatigue (CRF) compared to placebo during active treatment (Barton et al., 2010; Barton et al., 2013). *Panax ginseng* (Korean ginseng), which contains a similar ginsenoside profile to *P. quenquefolius* (Barton et al., 2013), was found to improve emotional functioning and decrease symptoms of fatigue, nausea, vomiting, dyspnea, anxiety and daytime somnolence, without impacting prognosis in a small study of women with ovarian cancer (Kim et al., 2017). Not all studies of ginseng have found benefit to energy (Yennurajalingam et al., 2017), which may reflect differences in ginseng species, extraction and processing methods, dosages, and length of intervention. Clinical and pre-clinical research demonstrates the ability of ginseng to down-regulate inflammatory pathways and modulate the HPA axis (Jin et al., 2010; Jung et al., 2011; Kang et al., 2011), which are known factors implicated in the pathogenesis of CRF (Bower et al., 2005).

Mistletoe (*Viscum album*) is a parasitic plant with a long history of use in cancer care. Mistletoe preparations contain various biologically active compounds including lectins, viscotoxins and polysaccharides which contribute to the immunomodulatory and cytotoxic actions of mistletoe (Marvibaigi et al., 2014). Injectable mistletoe extracts have been evaluated alongside conventional treatment for a variety of cancers, including breast (Troger et al., 2014), lung (Bar-Scla et al., 2013), colorectal (Bock et al., 2014) and gynaecological cancers (Ziegler and Grossarth-Maticek, 2010). In general, most studies show benefit for quality of life and side effect outcomes, results are mixed for survival and tumour response outcomes, and methodological concerns are common (Horneber et al., 2012). A 2009 systematic review looking specifically at survival outcomes in cancer patients treated with adjuvant mistletoe therapy found that there was a survival advantage associated with mistletoe, however, publication bias and heterogeneity in methodology were considered high and thus should be interpreted with caution (Ostermann et al., 2009). For breast cancer specifically, the evidence for mistletoe as quality of life support is fairly strong; the Society for Integrative Oncology clinical practice guideline for breast cancer (Greenlee et al., 2017) assigns a grade C for mistletoe, indicating it can be considered for use alongside conventional cancer treatments.

Mushroom extracts such as *Coriolus versicolor* (Turkey tail) and *Ganoderma lucidum* (Reishi) have promising emerging evidence for their role in cancer management; meta-analyses examining *C. versicolor* have reported improved five-year cancer survival rates (Eliza et al., 2012) while *G. lucidum* use alongside chemo/radiotherapy enhanced the likelihood of a positive response compared to chemo/radiotherapy alone and demonstrated positive effects on immune function and quality of life (Jin et al., 2016). However, many of the RCTs in both meta-analyses have small samples sizes and weak methodological quality. Mushroom polysaccharides have immunomodulatory effects, which is one of the main reasons for their use (Cui and Chisti, 2003; Sohretoglu and Huang, 2017). Both mushrooms have good safety profiles as discussed in the systematic reviews.

Melatonin, a hormone produced by the pineal gland, has been studied with positive outcomes for reducing pre-operative anxiety (Hansen et al., 2015), the side effects of chemo/radiotherapy, and overall survival outcomes for individuals with mixed solid tumours (Seely et al., 2012). A meta-analysis found that pre-operative administration of melatonin reduced pre-operative anxiety equally as effectively as midazolam, and the quality of RCTs included was considered high (Hansen et al., 2015). The molecular mechanisms of melatonin are broad and complex; current pre-clinical evidence suggests melatonin may evoke its impact through modulation of inflammation, oxidation, angiogenesis, and immune function among others (Reiter et al., 2017).

Clinical practice guidelines have been developed by the Society for Integrative Oncology for breast cancer (Greenlee et al., 2017), lung cancer (Deng et al., 2013), and integrative oncology in general (Deng et al., 2009). With continued research on integrative therapies, there will hopefully be sufficient evidence in the future for guidelines to be expanded to other cancer types to enhance and encourage the use of evidence-based CIM in women's cancer management plans.

## Role of CIM in stress management in women's cancer

There are several factors that have been identified as risk factors in women's cancers such as the family history, presence of high-susceptibility genes, excessive body weight and chronic stress (Cormanique et al., 2015). Focusing on the chronic stress and implementing CIM practices to assist the management of this type of stress may assist in the prevention of cancer development, recurrence and longevity.

The majority of research on psychological stress and women's cancer focuses on patients who have recently been diagnosed, are currently receiving treatment, are post treatment and/or those with advanced cancer/palliative care (Tschuschke et al., 2017). These studies have shown that developing active coping behaviours have more beneficial effects compared to passive anxious coping behaviours (ibid.). CIM practitioners can assist by educating patients on active coping behaviours as well as implementing cortisol-lowering herbal medicine, such as *Withania somnifera* (Choudhary et al., 2017) or nutrients that support the stress response such as magnesium (Tarasov et al., 2015).

Research on psychological stress and the development of breast cancer is limited but growing. The mechanism of action of psychological distress is that chronic exposure (beyond 6 months) can impair the immune function and increase the development of abnormal cells, which in turn predisposes an individual to the development of cancer (Verburg-van Kemenade et al., 2017) It has been found that exposure to a chronic stressor in the last five years preceding diagnosis is a risk factor for cancer development (Ozkan et al., 2017). A study on chronic psychological distress and its impact on the development of aggressive breast cancer (n = 34 women) found that chronic psychological distress constituted a considerable risk factor for weight gain and the development of aggressive tumours in women diagnosed with breast cancer (Cormanique et al., 2015). Interestingly, this work conducted in Brazil also found 73 per cent of the participants attributed this stress to the development of their cancer (ibid.). A case-control study examining lifestyle and psychological distress on the development of early onset breast cancer found that besides age at first birth, history of breast cancer in an immediate family member and history of genital surgery, lifestyle and psychological stress play an important role in the risk of breast cancer development (Li et al., 2016).

Overall, focusing on stress management and psychological factors may assist in decreasing the development of cancer. CIM practices that treat and manage frequent depression and negative emotional experiences in addition to balancing neuroendocrine hormones in women, have the potential to reduce the odds of cancer development (Satija and Bhatnagar, 2017). Addressing biopsychosocial factors in health care plays an important role in the prevention of cancer as well as potentially decreasing recurrence. CIM practices, such as yoga, acupuncture, T'ai Chi, qigong, massage, spiritual or energy therapies (Satija and Bhatnagar, 2017), in addition to diet, exercise, nutritional or herbal medicine supplementation (Greenlee et al., 2017) have the capacity and research support to indicate their use in stress reduction and possible cancer prevention.

## Cancer survivorship and CIM

From 1975–1977, women diagnosed with cancer were found to have a 55.9 per cent (in the USA) or 34 per cent (in England) chance of surviving five years. In 2006–2012, females now have a 68.36 per cent (in the USA) or 59 per cent (England) chance of surviving 5 years after diagnosis (Economist Intelligence Unit, 2017). The survival rate for breast cancer in America, as of 2013, has a 89.7 per cent survival rate (ibid.). This growing population of cancer survivors has brought with it a wave of survivorship care plans (Spronk et al., 2017). Given the increasing number of both long-term and newly diagnosed cancer survivors, attention to their special health needs and to reducing their risk of recurrence is critical.

The medical health system now recognizes that survivorship is an important phase of the cancer journey with an acknowledgement that the cancer experience does not end with the close of treatment (ibid.). Ongoing challenges in physical, psychological, social and economic health can compromise recovery and well-being in survivorship (ibid.). Despite the fact that cancer survivors have significant health needs, a variety of surveys indicate that anywhere from 30–60 per cent of cancer survivors feel their special health needs are not being met (Boyes et al., 2012; McDowell et al., 2010). In the physical realm, 80 per cent of patients treated with chemotherapy experience fatigue and up to 90 per cent of those treated with radiation experience fatigue (Hofman et al., 2007). Sleep disturbances affect between 30 per cent and 75 per cent of people diagnosed with cancer (Fiorentino, 2007). Up to 75 per cent of people diagnosed with cancer experience cognitive impairment during or after treatment and in 35 per cent of those cases, it can persist for months or even years after treatment is over (Janelsins et al., 2011; Wang et al., 2015). From a psychological standpoint, up to 70 per cent of cancer survivors report "clinically significant levels" of fear of recurrence and this is true even when actual recurrence risk is low (Butow et al., 2013).

To assist female cancer survivors recover their health following treatment and reduce the risk of recurrence, more emphasis needs to be placed on strategies associated with impactful lifestyle areas (Denlinger et al., 2014). These areas include diet, exercise, environmental toxin exposure, stress management, and psychosocial wellness. Numerous studies now demonstrate that engagement in a healthy lifestyle that includes a whole foods unprocessed diet, weight control, smoking cessation, and physical activity can counter some of the adverse effects of treatment and reduce recurrence risk while enhancing overall quality of life (Vijayvergia, 2015). These are areas which are solidly within the expertise of the CIM practitioner (Viscuse et al., 2017), thus directing cancer survivors into the care of CIM practitioners represents an ideal clinical path. Population-based studies report that cancer survivors are avid users of CIM approaches with usage rates ranging from 65 per cent (ever used) to 40 per cent (used in the past year) (Mao et al., 2011) and the usage rates do not reduce over time (Sohl et al., 2014). Cancer survivors are typically highly motivated (Vijayvergia and Denlinger, 2015) and, when given the right tools and guidance, can become proactive in their recovery and healing process.

## Conclusion

CIM can and currently does play a major role in the prevention, as an adjunct to treatment, survival and quality of life for women who have cancer or are at risk. The integration of CIM in the oncology arena is still in its infancy stages but integrative oncology is slowly becoming more accepted by the mainstream oncology health professionals. Many challenges still lie ahead, in particular with communication, understanding of the benefits of integration and true integration of CIM in the oncology world. Patient CIM use and openness are the key to bringing all health professionals together for the best benefit of women with cancer.

## Notes

1   A healthy dietary pattern is characterized by consumption of higher portions of fruit and vegetables, wholegrain foods, poultry, fish, lower consumption of red meat and fatty foods, low consumption of salt, sugar, coffee, sugary drinks and alcohol.
2   A Western-style diet is characterized by consumption of excessive amount of refined and processed foods, alcohol, salt, red meat and processed meat, high refined grains, high sugar drinks, full fat dairy foods, low fruit and vegetable intake and low fibre intake.

## References

Bar-Sela, G., Wollner, M., Hammer, L. et al. 2013. Mistletoe as complementary treatment in patients with advanced non-small-cell lung cancer treated with carboplatin-based combinations: a randomised phase II study. *European Journal of Cancer*, 49, 1058–64.

Barton, D. L., Liu, H., Dakhil, S. R. et al. 2013. Wisconsin ginseng (Panax quinquefolius) to improve cancer-related fatigue: a randomized, double-blind trial, N07C2. *Journal of National Cancer Institute*, 105, 1230–8.

Barton, D. L., Soori, G. S., Bauer, B. A. et al. 2010. Pilot study of Panax quinquefolius (American ginseng) to improve cancer-related fatigue: a randomized, double-blind, dose-finding evaluation: NCCTG trial N03CA. *Supportive Care in Cancer*, 18, 179–87.

Benetou V, T. A., Orfanos, P. et al. 2008. Conformity to traditional Mediterranean diet and cancer incidence: the Greek EPIC cohort. *British Journal of Cancer*, 99, 191.

Bidoli E, F. S., Talamini, R. et al. 1992. Food consumption and cancer of the colon and rectum in northeastern Italy. *International Journal of Cancer*, 50, 223–9.

Bock, P. R., Hanisch, J., Matthes, H. and Zanker, K. S. 2014. Targeting inflammation in cancer-related-fatigue: a rationale for mistletoe therapy as supportive care in colorectal cancer patients. *Inflammation and Allergy: Drug Targets*, 13, 105–11.

Bower, J. E., Ganz, P. A. and Aziz, N. 2005. Altered cortisol response to psychologic stress in breast cancer survivors with persistent fatigue. *Psychosomatic Medicine*, 67, 277–80.

Boyes A. W., D'Este, C., and Zucca, A. C. 2012. Prevalence and correlates of cancer survivors' supportive care needs 6 months after diagnosis: a population-based cross-sectional study. *BioMed Central*, 12, 150.

Bradbury, K. A. P. and Key, T. J. 2014. Fruit, vegetable, and fiber intake in relation to cancer risk: findings from the European Prospective Investigation into Cancer and Nutrition (EPIC). *American Journal of Clin Nutrition*, 100(suppl), 394S–8S.

Butow P. N., Smith A. B. et al. 2013. Conquer fear: protocol of a randomized controlled trial of a psychological intervention to reduce fear of cancer recurrence. *BMC Cancer*, 13, 201.

Campbell, P. T., Patel, A. V., Newton, C. C., Jacobs, E. J. and Gapstur, S. M. 2013. Associations of recreational physical activity and leisure time spent sitting with colorectal cancer survival. *Journal of Clinical Oncology*, 31, 876–85.

Cannioto, R., Kelemen, L. E. et al. 2016. Recreational physical inactivity and mortality in women with invasive epithelial ovarian cancer: evidence from the Ovarian Cancer Association Consortium. *British Journal of Cancer*, 115, 95–101.

Carlson, L. E., Zelinski, E., Toivonen, K. et al. 2017. Mind-body therapies in cancer: what is the latest evidence? *Current Oncology Reports*, 19, 67.

Chen, L., Lin, C. C., Huang, T. W. et al. 2017. Effect of acupuncture on aromatase inhibitor-induced arthralgia in patients with breast cancer: a meta-analysis of randomized controlled trials. *Breast*, 33, 132–8.

Chen, L., Ye, R., Zhang, W. et al. 2016. Endocrine disruption throughout the hypothalamus-pituitary-gonadal-liver (HPGL) axis in marine medaka (oryzias melastigma) chronically exposed to the antifouling and chemopreventive agent, 3,3′-diindolylmethane (DIM). *Chemical Research in Toxicology*, 29, 1020–8.

Choudhary, D., Bhattacharyya, S. and Joshi, K. 2017. Body weight management in adults under chronic stress through treatment with ashwagandha root extract: a double-blind, randomized, placebo-controlled trial. *Journal of Evidence-Based Complementary Alternative Medicine*, 22, 96–106.

Cormanique, T. F., Almeida, L. E., Rech, C. A. et al. 2015. Chronic psychological stress and its impact on the development of aggressive breast cancer. *Einstein (São Paulo)*, 13, 352–6.

Cramer, H., Lauche, R., Klose, P. et al. 2017. Yoga for improving health-related quality of life, mental health and cancer-related symptoms in women diagnosed with breast cancer. *Cochrane Database of Systematic Reviews*, 1, Cd010802.

Cui, J. and Chisti, Y. 2003. Polysaccharopeptides of Coriolus versicolor: physiological activity, uses, and production. *Biotechnologyl Advances*, 21, 109–22.

Deng, G. E., Cohen, L. et al. 2009. Evidence-based clinical practice guidelines for integrative oncology: complementary therapies and botanicals. *Journal of Society for Integrative Oncology*, 7, 85–120.

Deng, G. E., Rausch, S. M., Jones, L. W. et al. 2013. *Complementary Therapies and Integrative Medicine in Lung Cancer: Diagnosis and Management of Lung Cancer*, 3rd ed: American College of Chest Physicians evidence-based clinical practice guidelines. *Chest*, 143, e420S–e436S.

Denlinger, C. L. J., Are, M. et al. 2014. Survivorship: nutrition and weight management, version 2.2014: clinical practice guidelines in oncology. *Journal of the National Comprehensive Cancer Network*, 12, 1396–406.

Dibble, S. L., Luce, J., Cooper, B. A. et al. 2007. Acupressure for chemotherapy-induced nausea and vomiting: a randomized clinical trial. *Oncology Nursing Forum*, 34, 813–20.

Economist Intelligence Unit. 2017. Cancer survivorship: a portrait. [Online]. Available at: www.cancersurvivorship.eiu.com (accessed 19 December 2017).

Eliza, W. L., Fai, C. K. and Chung, L. P. 2012. Efficacy of Yun Zhi (Coriolus versicolor) on survival in cancer patients: systematic review and meta-analysis. *Recent Patents on Inflammation and Allergy Drug Discovery*, 6, 78–87.

Fan, Y., Jin, X., Man, C., Gao, Z. and Wang, X. 2017. Meta-analysis of the association between the inflammatory potential of diet and colorectal cancer risk. *Oncotarget*, 8, 59592–600.

Fiorentino, L, 2007. Sleep dysfunction in patients with cancer. *Current Treatment Options in Neurology*, 9, 337–46.

Gann P, C. R., Gapstur S.M. et al. 2003. The effects of a low-fat/high-fiber diet on sex hormone levels and menstrual cycling in premenopausal women: a 12-month randomized trial (the diet and hormone study). *Cancer*, 98, 1870–9.

Greenlee, H., Dupont-Reyes, M. J., Balneaves, L. G. et al. 2017. Clinical practice guidelines on the evidence-based use of integrative therapies during and after breast cancer treatment. *CA: A Cancer Journal for Clinicians*, 67, 194–232.

Greenlee, H., Ergas, I. J. et al. 2009. Complementary and alternative therapy use before and after breast cancer diagnosis: the Pathways Study. *Breast Cancer Research Treatment*, 117, 653–65.

Haller, H., Winkler, M. M., Klose, P. et al. 2017. Mindfulness-based interventions for women with breast cancer: an updated systematic review and meta-analysis. *Acta Oncologica*, 56, 1665–76.

Hansen, M. V., Halladin, N. L., Rosenberg, J., Gogenur, I. and Moller, A. M. 2015. Melatonin for pre- and postoperative anxiety in adults. *Cochrane Database of Systematic Reviews*, Cd009861.

Hedderson, M., Neuhouser, M. L. et al. 2004. Sex differences in motives for use of complementary and alternative medicine among cancer patients. *Alternative Therapies in Health and Medicine*, 10, 58–64.

Hofman, M., Figueroa-Moseley, C. D. et al. 2007. Cancer-related fatigue: the scale of the problem. *The Oncologist*, 12, 4–10.

Horneber, M, B. G., Dennert, G., Less, D., Ritter, E., and Zwahlen, M. 2012. How many cancer patients use complementary and alternative medicine? *Integrative Cancer Therapies*, 11, 187–203.

Irwin, M. L, McTiernan, A. et al. 2008. Influence of pre- and postdiagnosis physical activity on mortality in breast cancer survivors: the health, eating, activity, and lifestyle study. *Journal of Clinical Oncology*, 20, 3958–64.

Janelsins, M., Mohile, S. G. et al. 2011. An update on cancer- and chemotherapy-related cognitive dysfunction: current status. *Seminars in Oncology*, 38, 431–8.

Jin, X., Sze, D. M., Chan, G. C. T. 2016. Ganoderma lucidum (Reishi mushroom) for cancer treatment. *Cochrane Database of Systematic Reviews*.

Jin, Y., Hofseth, A. B., Cui, X. et al. 2010. American ginseng suppresses colitis through p53-mediated apoptosis of inflammatory cells. *Cancer Prevention Research (Phila)*, 3, 339–47.

Jung, H. L., Kwak, H. E., Kim, S. S.,et al. 2011. Effects of Panax ginseng supplementation on muscle damage and inflammation after uphill treadmill running in humans. *American Journal of Chinese Medicine*, 39, 441–50.

Kang, A., Hao, H., Zheng, X. et al. 2011. Peripheral anti-inflammatory effects explain the ginsenosides paradox between poor brain distribution and anti-depression efficacy. *Journal of Neuroinflammation*, 8, 100.

Kim, H. S., Kim, M. K., Lee, M. et al. 2017. Effect of red ginseng on genotoxicity and health-related quality of life after adjuvant chemotherapy in patients with epithelial ovarian cancer: a randomized, double blind, placebo-controlled trial. *Nutrients*, 9.

Krohn, M., Listing, M., Tjahjono, G. et al. 2011. Depression, mood, stress, and Th1/Th2 immune balance in primary breast cancer patients undergoing classical massage therapy. *Supportive Care in Cancer*, 19, 1303–11.

Kwon, Y. 2014. Effect of soy isoflavones on the growth of human breast tumors: findings from preclinical studies. *Food Science & Nutrition*, 2, 613–22.

Lee, A. C. S. and Fan, L. T. 2015. *Stimulation of the Wrist Acupuncture Point PC6 for Preventing Postoperative Nausea and Vomiting.*, Chichester: John Wiley & Sons, Ltd.

Levi, F,. P. C., Lucchini, F., and La Vecchia, C. 2001. Dietary fibre and the risk of colorectal cancer. *European Journal of Cancer Prevention*, 37, 2091–6.

Li, P., Huang, J., Wu, H., et al. 2016. Impact of lifestyle and psychological stress on the development of early onset breast cancer. *Medicine (Baltimore)*, 95, e5529.

Lopresti, A. L. 2017. Cognitive behaviour therapy and inflammation: a systematic review of its relationship and the potential implications for the treatment of depression. *Australian and New Zealand Journal of Psychiatry*, 51, 565–82.

Mao, J., Healy, K. E. et al. 2011. Complementary and alternative medicine use among cancer survivors: a population-based study. *Journal of Cancer Survivorship*, 5, 8–17.

Marvibaigi, M., Supriyanto, E., Amini, N., Abdul Majid, F. A. and Jaganathan, S. K. 2014. Preclinical and clinical effects of mistletoe against breast cancer. *BioMed Research International*, 2014, 785479.

McDowell, M. E., Ferguson, M. et al. 2010. Predictors of change in unmet care needs in cancer. *Psycho-Oncology*, 19, 508–16.

Molassiotis, A., Helin, A. M., Dabbour, R. and Hummerston, S. 2007. The effects of P6 acupressure in the prophylaxis of chemotherapy-related nausea and vomiting in breast cancer patients. *Complementary Therapies in Medicine*, 15, 3–12.

Muc-Wierzgoń, M., Dzięgielewska-Gęsiak, S. et al. 2014. Specific metabolic biomarkers as risk and prognostic factors in colorectal cancer. *World Journal of Gastroenterology*, 20, 9759–74.

Muscaritoli, M., Amabile, M. I. and Molfino, A. 2016. Foods and their components promoting gastrointestinal cancer. *Current Opinion in Clinical Nutrition and Metabolic Care*, 19(5), 1.

Narita, S., Inoue, M., Saito, E. et al. 2017. Dietary fiber intake and risk of breast cancer defined by estrogen and progesterone receptor status: the Japan Public Health Center-based Prospective Study. *Cancer Causes Control*, 28, 569–578.

National Cancer Institute. 2017. *Cancer Stat Facts: Female Breast Cancer.* Available at: www.cancer.gov (accessed 19 December 2017).

National Institute of Environmental Health Sciences. 2017. Endocrine disruptors fact sheet. Available at: www.niehs.nih.gov/health/materials/endocrine_disruptors

Nechuta, S. J., Chen Wy, C. B., et al. 2012. Soy food intake after diagnosis of breast cancer and survival: an in-depth analysis of combined evidence from cohort studies of US and Chinese women. *American Journal of Clinical Nutrition*, 96, 123–132.

Ostermann, T., Raak, C. and Bussing, A. 2009. Survival of cancer patients treated with mistletoe extract (Iscador): a systematic literature review. *BMC Cancer*, 9, 451.

Ozkan, M., Yildirim, N., Disci, R. et al. 2017. Roles of biopsychosocial factors in the development of breast cancer. *European Journal of Breast Health*, 13, 206–212.

Pascoe, M. C., Thompson, D. R. and Ski, C. F. 2017. Yoga, mindfulness-based stress reduction and stress-related physiological measures: a meta-analysis. *Psychoneuroendocrinology*, 86, 152–168.

Perduca, V., Omichessan, H., Baglietto, L. and Severi, G. 2018. Mutational and epigenetic signatures in cancer tissue linked to environmental exposures and lifestyle. *Current Opinion in Oncology*, 30, 61–67.

Reiter, R. J., Rosales-Corral, S. A., Tan, D. X. et al. 2017. Melatonin, a full service anti-cancer agent: inhibition of initiation, progression and metastasis. *International Journal of Molecular Science*, 18.

Rithirangsriroj, K., Manchana, T. and Akkayagorn, L. 2015. Efficacy of acupuncture in prevention of delayed chemotherapy induced nausea and vomiting in gynecologic cancer patients. *Gynecologic Oncology*, 136, 82–86.

Romagnolo, D. F. and Selmin, O. I. 2017. Mediterranean diet and prevention of chronic diseases. *Nutrition Today*, 52, 208–222.

Satija, A. and Bhatnagar, S. 2017. Complementary therapies for symptom management in cancer patients. *Indian Journal of Palliative Care*, 23, 468–479.

Seely, D., Wu, P., Fritz, H.,et al. 2012. Melatonin as adjuvant cancer care with and without chemotherapy: a systematic review and meta-analysis of randomized trials. *Integrative Cancer Therapies*, 11, 293–303.

Segal, R., Zwaal, C., Green, E. et al. 2017. Exercise for people with cancer: a systematic review. *Current Oncology*, 24, e290–e315.

Shapira, N. 2017. The potential contribution of dietary factors to breast cancer prevention. *European Journal of Cancer Prevention*, 26, 385–395.

Shin, E-S., Lee, S-H. et al. 2016. Massage with or without aromatherapy for symptom relief in people with cancer. *Cochrane Database of Systematic Reviews*.

Sohl, S.J., Birdee, G. et al. 2014. Characteristics associated with the use of complementary health approaches among long-term cancer survivors. *Supportive Care in Cancer*, 22, 927–936.

Sohretoglu, D. and Huang, S. 2017. Ganoderma lucidum polysaccharides as an anti-cancer agent. *Anticancer Agents in Medicinal Chemistry*, 17. doi: 10.2174/18715206176661 71113121246

Spronk, I., Korevaar, J. C., Schellevis, F. G. et al. 2017. Evidence-based recommendations on care for breast cancer survivors for primary care providers: a review of evidence-based breast cancer guidelines. *BMJ Open*, 7, e015118.

Stagl, J. M., Lechner, S. C., Carver, C. S. et al. 2015. A randomized controlled trial of cognitive-behavioral stress management in breast cancer: survival and recurrence at 11-year follow-up. *Breast Cancer Research and Treatment*, 154, 319–328.

Sun, L., Subar, A. F., Bosire, C. et al. 2017. Dietary flavonoid intake reduces the risk of head and neck but not esophageal or gastric cancer in US men and women. *Journal of Nutrition*, 147, 1729–1738.

Tarasov, E. A., Blinov, D. V., Zimovina, U. V. and Sandakova, E. A. 2015. Magnesium deficiency and stress: issues of their relationship, diagnostic tests, and approaches to therapy. *Ter Arkh*, 87, 114–122.

Troger, W., Zdrale, Z., Tisma, N. and Matijasevic, M. 2014. Additional therapy with a mistletoe product during adjuvant chemotherapy of breast cancer patients improves quality of life: an open randomized clinical pilot trial. *Evidence-Based Complementary Alternative Medicine*, 2014, 430518.

Tschuschke, V., Karadaglis, G., Evangelou, K., Grafin Von Schweinitz, C. and Schwickerath, J. 2017. Psychological stress and coping resources during primary systemic therapy for breast cancer. results of a prospective study. *Geburtshilfe Frauenheilkunde*, 77, 158-168.

Verburg-Van Kemenade, B. M., Cohen, N. and Chadzinska, M. 2017. Neuroendocrine-immune interaction: evolutionarily conserved mechanisms that maintain allostasis in an ever-changing environment. *Developmental and Comparative Immunology*, 66, 2–23.

Vijayvergia N, D. C. and Denlinger, C. S.2015. Lifestyle factors in cancer survivorship: where we are and where we are headed. *Journal of Personalized Medicine*, 5, 243–263.

Viscuse, P. V., Price, K., Millstine, D. et al. 2017. Integrative medicine in cancer survivors. *Current Opinion in Oncology*, 29, 235–242.

Wai., F. K. 2005. National Center for Complementary and Alternative Medicine website. *Journal of the Medical Library Association*, 93, 410.

Wang, H. F., Yao, A. L., Sun, Y. Y. and Zhang, A. H. 2017. Empirically derived dietary patterns and ovarian cancer risk: a meta-analysis. *European Journal of Cancer Prevention*, doi: 10.1097/CEJ.0000000000000367.

Wang, X. W. B., Saligan, L. et al. 2015. Chemobrain: a critical review and causal hypothesis of link between cytokines and epigenetic reprogramming associated with chemotherapy. *Cytokine*, 72, 86–96.

WHO (World Health Organization) 2017a. Breast cancer. Available at: www.who.int/cancer/detection/breastcancer/en/ (accessed 8 November 2017).

WHO (World Health Organization ) 2017b. Cancer. Available at: www.who.int/cancer/en/ (accessed 8 November 2017).

Witt, C. B. L., Cardoso, M.J. et al. 2017. A comprehensive definition for integrative oncology. *JNCI Monographs*, 2017.

Xiao, F., Song, X., Chen, Q. et al. 2017. Effectiveness of psychological interventions on depression in patients after breast cancer surgery: a meta-analysis of randomized controlled trials. *Clinical Breast Cancer*, 17, 171–179.

Yennurajalingam, S., Tannir, N. M., Williams, J. L. et al. 2017. A double-blind, randomized, placebo-controlled trial of panax ginseng for cancer-related fatigue in patients with advanced cancer. *Journal of the National Comprehensive Cancer Network*, 15, 1111–1120.

Zhang, Y., Lin, L., Li, H., Hu, Y. and Tian, L. 2017. Effects of acupuncture on cancer-related fatigue: a meta-analysis. *Supportive Care in Cancer*, 26(2), 415–425.

Ziegler, R. and Grossarth-Maticek, R. 2010. Individual patient data meta-analysis of survival and psychosomatic self-regulation from published prospective controlled cohort studies for long-term therapy of breast cancer patients with a mistletoe preparation (iscador). *Evidence-Based Complementary Alternative Medicine*, 7, 157–166.

# 6   The use of self-care practices and products by women with chronic illness

## A case study of older women with osteoarthritis and osteoporosis

*Jon Adams, Jason Prior, David Sibbritt,*
*Irena Connon, Roger Dunston,*
*Erica McIntyre and Romy Lauche*

### Introduction

This chapter examines the use of complementary and integrative medicine (CIM) self-care practices and products with reference to women with chronic illness. Introducing a case study of women with osteoarthritis and osteoporosis – drawing upon the first focused empirical inquiry of a large sample of older women with either of these two conditions – the chapter explores the significance of the self-care concept in helping to understand significant dimensions of CIM use and interpret the actions of CIM users.

It is posited that reframing some aspects of CIM consumption as self-care behaviours and practices provides an excellent opportunity to reinvigorate CIM scholarship. This conceptualisation is also a powerful tool in gaining further insights into the role and consequences of CIM use in supporting women with chronic illness, highlighting a number of barriers, challenges and enablers to women achieving optimal relief from symptoms and a status of positive health (which may otherwise not be imagined or realised) and ultimately helping facilitate and encourage co-ordinated, effective and safe patient care based upon best knowledge of *all* practices and behaviours such women engage in to seek help and support. The chapter first sets the broader scene of a fast-growing chronic illness crisis and presents the associated burdens and the specific location of and issues for women within this crisis. Attention then turns to a concurrent trend – the growing popularity of CIM. More specifically, the focus is upon the rise of a sub-field of CIM practices and product use that can be conceptualised as constituting self-care and, until relatively recently, one that has been a hidden aspect of CIM neglected by both academics and many at the grass-roots level of women's health care practice. Introducing the case study of osteoarthritis and osteoporosis via new empirical data analysis from a large-scale survey of Australian women, the chapter reveals how CIM self-care shares certain particular features that not only identify its investigation of elevated scholarly significance but also poses a number of unique challenges and barriers to the provision of optimal health care provision for women with one of a vast range of chronic illnesses. As we argue in the conclusion, such challenges are of more than just the concern of CIM-focused users and should be an area of interest and engagement to all providing and facilitating health care to women with chronic illness, especially those who are more traditionally associated with the formal conventional health care system and medicine.

## The rise and burden of chronic illness and (older) women

Chronic illness – including a vast range of conditions such as asthma, stroke, diabetes, hypertension and other cardiovascular disease, depression and other affective disorders – lies at the heart of a fast-growing crisis for all health care systems around the world (WHO, 2017).

The number of Australians aged 65 and over will double in the next 30 years and rates of chronic illness increase significantly with age (AIHW, 2011). More than 15 million Australians are directly affected by at least one chronic illness (ibid.). The already large burden of chronic illness – currently directly responsible for nearly 80 per cent of the total burden of illness and injury – is set to grow dramatically with projections suggesting chronic illness will account for nearly half of all deaths and forms of disability in Australia by 2020 (Aspin et al., 2010). Chronic illness has profound impacts on daily living (Bury, 1982) with detrimental effects upon people's social, physical and psychological functioning and quality of life (Gunn et al., 2012). Research shows that despite best efforts to publicly fund essential care and support, many Australian households experience extensive economic hardship as a result of out-of-pocket expenses associated with chronic illnesses (Essue et al., 2011; Jan et al., 2012). This completes a cycle in which poor health leads to poverty, which then leads to poorer health.

We know that older women are over-represented in the ageing population, experience symptoms of chronic illness differently to men (O'Neill & Morrow, 2001), and have specific health needs (often not met by formal expert-led care) (Feldman et al., 2002). Furthermore, older women are significantly disadvantaged. Entrenched social and health inequalities, particularly related to employment and salary, can also impact negatively upon older women (Beaglehole et al., 2007). All these circumstances highlight the significance of studying and attempting to understand the complexities of women living with chronic illness in the community with a view to helping inform health services and a health system that can successfully address their ongoing needs and challenges. As discussed in the next section, such study and understanding necessitate an in-depth consideration of CIM, especially CIM self-care; behaviours and practices of consumption around seeking health and illness relief which have been largely neglected to date but which are increasingly being acknowledged as essential to ascertaining the broader picture of women's health and health care relating to chronic illness.

## The conventional medical response to chronic illness and the rise of CIM self-care

The conventional medical community has struggled to provide adequate care in the context of co-morbidity and the complexities of living with chronic illness (e.g. Jowsey et al., 2009; Jeon et al., 2010). While Australian initiatives such as the National Chronic Disease Strategy (Harris et al., 2008) have strongly advocated greater patient-centred and directed care (Kennedy et al., 2007; Greenhalgh, 2009), the extent to which these policies have been transferred into practice remains negligible. Furthermore, at a practice level, conventional health services – both practitioner-delivered and supported non-CIM forms of self-care (such as diet, exercise, non-prescription pain relief among others) – have largely failed to meet the complex needs of the chronically ill (Wellard, 2010).

Much work revealing the lived experiences of chronicity and the harsh impacts upon a sense of worth (Bury, 1982; Charmaz, 1983; Townsend et al., 2006), gendered identities (Werner et al., 2004), capacity to work (Blaxter, 1976; Walker, 2010) and role in the family (Corbin & Strauss, 1988; Gregory, 2005; Wilson, 2007) has been crucial to emphasising that chronic illness has slipped through the cracks of conventional medical health service delivery, including how those living with chronic illness struggle to gain the support and care they require (Charmaz, 1983; Corbin & Strauss, 1988).

Given the somewhat underwhelming achievements of conventional medical care to respond to the complexities and needs of those with chronic illness, it is perhaps unsurprising that CIM self-care may be occupying the vacuum in providing support for such sufferers. Indeed, CIM practitioners and practices have long been associated with promoting personalised care regimens and holistic support incorporating mind and body, rather than a focus upon disease/physiological pathology (Hill, 2003; Coulter, 2004). Indeed, recent research polemics/agenda positions (Adams et al., 2014; Adams, 2017) and empirical work (Thorne et al., 1997; Armstrong et al., 2011; Broom et al., 2012; Sibbritt et al., 2012; Adams et al., 2013) suggest that women use CIM self-care when conventional medical practitioners fail to relieve the burden of chronic illness for them and their families. Yet, as we will see in the following section, despite early signs of the prominence and potential of CIM self-care to recast roles and experiences for chronically ill women, there remains a fundamental lack of empirical investigation in this area. Furthermore, no work to date has provided in-depth examination of CIM self-care use among those women with osteoarthritis and osteoporosis. Before introducing the findings from the first such study, it is necessary to define CIM self-care and to outline why its study is so significant in conceptualising and charting women's CIM practice and use in the context of living with chronic illness.

## CIM self-care practices and products: definition, significance and as gendered social practice

### *A definition of CIM self-care*

As with all key concepts in health research, it is essential that we are clear about the definition of what is here referred to as CIM self-care. Self-care, in the context of this chapter, refers to activities undertaken for 'enhancing health, preventing disease, limiting illness, and restoring health' (WHO, 2009), principally or solely directed by the individual with minimal or no practitioner involvement. While self-care more broadly includes non-CIM activities such as exercise, diet and non-prescription pain relief, CIM self-care practices and products include such things as meditation, yoga, mindfulness, and herbal and naturopathic medicines. CIM self-care constitutes the bulk of self-care in Australia (Harris et al., 2012), and represents the single largest area of modern CIM consumption (Xue et al., 2007; Reid et al., 2016).

Importantly, CIM self-care use is located *in the community* and is primarily covert in nature – until now hidden from the core concerns of the vast majority of health scholars focused upon chronic illness as well as escaping the gaze and attention of many in the formal conventional health care system providing patient management for the chronically ill (Adams, 2017). CIM self-care is essentially the 'back stage' of chronic illness care; unexplored, unregulated and lacking critical examination.

### *CIM self-care as gendered practice*

CIM self-care use is particularly interesting with regards to women and women's health for a number of reasons. CIM use generally is much higher among women, and this has been linked to the potential 'affinity' of CIM with feminine ideas about the body, subjectivity and closeness to 'nature' (Sointu, 2006; Nissen, 2011). CIM practices, it has been argued, may enable some women to perform and embody ideas such as self-determination and self-actualisation (McLaughlin et al., 2012); aspects not often associated with conventional medical care. CIM practices, including CIM self-care, may promote divergent ideas around self-help and lay expertise, potentially enhancing a sense of agency and autonomy within the context of health, illness and well-being (Sointu, 2006; Broom, 2009). Indeed, one of the key features of CIM self-care activities is that the woman is in control of not only the information and resources available regarding practices and products but also the fundamental direction and character of her care. While professionals often instruct and support conventional medical self-care activities (i.e. providing encouragement and a framework for activities undertaken in the community that supplement a conventional medical paradigm, such as diet and exercise regimens), CIM self-care involves self-prescribing, self-instructing and an individually-driven therapeutic regimen and culture whereby women can tailor their approach according to their subjective experience. This fundamentally alters the philosophy and character of care, potentially allowing much greater agency and autonomy (Bishop & Yardley, 2004), but also introducing significant uncertainty and risk (Broom et al., 2014).

### The significance of CIM self-care

CIM self-care in many ways reflects a radical reframing of health and illness around the individual as the decision-maker, as the agent of change, and as responsible for the development of more personalised therapeutic regimens. Indeed, the importance of CIM self-care both as a substantive topic and a focus for investigation among women with chronic illness is essentially four-fold. We outline and discuss each of these issues below.

- *Disconnect with conventional medical care.* CIM self-care represents a set of practices disconnected from conventional medical care. Whereas conventional medical practitioners support various non-CIM self-care activities and in many cases develop referral networks with CIM practitioners (located beyond the formal health care system), CIM self-care remains marginalised from the woman-conventional medical interface in chronic illness care. This creates the potential for fragmentation in the woman's care, miscommunication, conflict between regimens, and, practitioners and women working at cross-purposes. All these issues culminate in an environment which can fuel and exacerbate some of the potential direct and indirect risks associated with women's use of practices and products beyond the gaze of conventional medical providers.
- *Philosophically divergent from conventional medical approaches.* CIM self-care may draw upon Eastern philosophical traditions or focus on the wider significance of illness and well-being, including the mind-body relationship. This includes a unique role for the woman in treatment choice, promoting flexibility over the mix and style of treatment and practice undertaken.
- *Beyond the control of the state or health practitioners.* CIM self-care by its very nature, as community-based, unregulated activities undertaken beyond the formal health care system, is significantly exposed to social disadvantage. Much CIM self-care (products especially) requires extensive out-of-pocket costs and also discriminates in terms of cultural capital and access/ participation, and the degree to which such social advantage and disadvantage may feed into this hidden sector of health seeking remains an issue worthy of much research resource.
- *Potentially enhancing chronic illness care.* Finally, not all circumstances surrounding CIM self-care use among women with chronic illness necessarily constitute a challenge or barrier to effective care. Indeed, CIM self-care activities may in many cases hold much potential and opportunity for helping women cope better with chronic illness. It is a potentially under-recognised means of enhancing chronic illness care for women and the important point is not so much its existence but the degree to which it can and will be subject to critical evidence-based evaluation and assessment.

As a means of extending the empirical literature of CIM self-care use in chronic illness, this chapter now turns attention to describing the first study to examine the prevalence of CIM self-care use among a large sample of women with osteoarthritis and osteoporosis.

## A case study: CIM self-care use among 797 women with osteoarthritis or osteoporosis

### *Osteoarthritis background*

Osteoarthritis (OA) is one of the most common chronic diseases affecting the elderly (Guccione et al., 1994). It is characterised by destruction of the cartilage that overlies the ends of the bones in the joints, in addition to underlying bony changes at the joint margins (Altman et al., 1986). The primary symptoms include joint pain and stiffness, often with severe functional impairment in daily life (Reginster, 2002).

Joint replacements are usually considered the last resorts for individuals diagnosed with osteoarthritis. The majority of patients with light to moderate symptoms will receive symptomatic treatment instead, mostly in form of use of oral and topical nonsteroidal anti-inflammatory drugs (NSAIDs). Guidelines also strongly recommend physical activity to improve pain and joint function (Hochberg et al., 2012), and to support weight loss which is essential as overweight and obesity contribute to almost 50 per cent of the total burden of osteoarthritis (Australian Institute of Health and Welfare, 2017).

Osteoporosis is a disease characterised by reduced bone density and quality, weakening the skeleton and increasing the risk of fractures, particularly at the hip, spine or wrist (Kanis, Melton, Christiansen, Johnston, & Khaltaev, 1994). As per the World Health Organization guidelines, osteoporosis is defined via bone mineral density, and individuals are diagnosed with osteoporosis when they have a bone mineral density at the hip and/or lumbar spine at or below 2.5 standard deviations below the average density of young healthy adults, and they are diagnosed with osteopenia when the bone mineral density is between 1.0 and 2.5 standard deviations below that of average healthy young adults (WHO, 1994). Approximately two-thirds of people over 50 years already have osteoporosis, osteopenia or poor bone health; and recent estimates for Australia also expect an increase in osteoporosis of 30 per cent until 2022 (Watts, Abimanyi-Ochom, & Sanders, 2013).

In order to improve bone health and prevent osteoporotic fractures, it is often recommended to use supplements such as vitamin D and calcium. Both vitamin D and calcium have known biologic effects on mineral homeostasis, and deficiencies in vitamin D and calcium have been associated with increased risk of fractures (LeBoff et al., 1999). In line with evidence, current guidelines, however, recommend supplementation only for institutionalised individuals, and those with known deficiencies (Avenell, Mak, & O'Connell, 2014; The Royal Australian College of General Practitioners & Osteoporosis Australia, 2017). Overall, supplementation of vitamin D and calcium appears to be common in elderly women, with 60.0 per cent of women over 65 years of age who have been diagnosed with osteoporosis using vitamin D and calcium supplementation on a daily basis (45 & Up study). Other preventive recommendations include exercise prescriptions, including resistance training and balance training exercises (The Royal Australian College of General Practitioners & Osteoporosis Australia, 2017) to improve bone structure, density and fracture resistance (Nikander et al., 2010; Howe et al., 2011). Balance training can also reduce the risk of falls in elderly individuals with poor balance (Sherrington et al., 2008).

Primary and secondary preventive drug treatment of osteoporosis includes bisphosphonates which can significantly increase bone mineral density, and reduce the risk of fractures in postmenopausal women with osteoporosis (Eriksen, Diez-Perez, & Boonen, 2014). Women taking bisphosphonates, however, may experience side effects, from gastrointestinal problems to musculoskeletal pain (Poole & Compston, 2012), leading to poor compliance (Silverman, Schousboe, & Gold, 2011), and strategies are needed to increase compliance to guarantee an optimal antifracture efficacy (Rabenda, Hiligsmann, & Reginster, 2009).

Hormone replacement therapy is further recommended for postmenopausal women, however the risk of adverse events associated with HRT need to be carefully weighed against potential benefits (The Royal Australian College of General Practitioners & Osteoporosis Australia, 2017).

*CIM for osteoporosis and osteoarthritis*

One CIM intervention with proven benefits for falls prevention is Tai Chi (Gillespie et al., 2012). Tai Chi, often referred to as shadow boxing, is a low-impact exercise originating in China. Tai Chi can easily be adapted for adults with physical limitations, such as individuals of residential-aged care facilities (Tsai et al., 2009). Tai Chi can improve pain, and quality of life in knee osteoarthritis (Lauche, Langhorst, Dobos, & Cramer, 2013) with similar benefits as physical therapy in OA of the knee (Wang et al., 2016), and it might help to maintain bone mineral density in postmenopausal women (Wayne et al., 2007), while at the same time having a very low risk profile (Wayne, Berkowitz, Litrownik, Buring, & Yeh, 2014).

There is also preliminary evidence for the efficacy of yoga in osteoarthritis, as such, it is included in current clinical practice guidelines (Brosseau et al., 2017). Contrary to Tai Chi, however, some yoga postures have the potential to aggravate joint problems, so its application needs to be considered carefully (Cramer, Ostermann, & Dobos, 2017).

Acupuncture is often used in osteoarthritis for pain management, with 7.7 per cent of women over 65 years with osteoarthritis reported consulting an acupuncturist in the last 12 months (45 & Up study). While research finds acupuncture only minimally effective for osteoarthritis of the knee (Manheimer et al., 2010), it is recommended conditionally for patients for chronic moderate to severe pain (Hochberg et al., 2012).

Physical therapies, including manual therapies, are recommended only in conjunction with supervised exercise (ibid.). While individual studies have indicated that massages may improve pain, joint function and well-being in knee osteoarthritis, a recent systematic review concluded that the evidence was inconclusive (French, Brennan, White, & Cusack, 2011).

Chondroitin and glucosamine are found naturally in the joint cartilage, and nutritional supplements are advertised to improve pain and function in osteo-arthritis, evidence, however, shows only small benefits over placebo (Towheed et al., 2005; Singh, Noorbaloochi, MacDonald, & Maxwell, 2015). While current guidelines explicitly recommend not using chondroitin and glucosamine (Hochberg et al., 2012), one in four women over 65 years with osteoarthritis reported the use of chondroitin and/or glucosamine on a daily basis (45 & Up study).

Several herbal therapies have been examined for osteoarthritis, including boswellia, curcuma, devil's claw and ginger. While oral herbal medicines are frequently used by individuals with arthritis (Yang, Sibbritt, & Adams, 2017), the evidence is still inconclusive for the majority of oral herbal preparations (Cameron & Chrubasik, 2014).

The quality and quantity of current research studies on topical herbal therapies are also insufficient (Cameron & Chrubasik, 2013), however, it seems that Arnica gel might improve OA symptoms as effectively as topical NSAID applications. Evidence for capsicum and ginger, on the other hand, were mostly negative.

Lastly, heat or cold application might be beneficial for OA pain, yet the lack of evidence renders any conclusion at this time. Preliminary evidence has been reported for ice-pack applications to reduce swelling and pain (Brosseau et al., 2003).

## Methods

### Sample

Data was obtained from a sub-study of the 45 and Up Study – the largest study of the healthy ageing population conducted in the Southern Hemisphere. The baseline questionnaire of the 45 and Up Study collected information from 266,848 men and women aged 45 and above who reside in the State of New South Wales, Australia (45 and Up Study Collaborators, 2008). Recruitment for the 45 and Up Study involved individuals aged 45 years and above and resident in the State of New South Wales randomly selected from the Department of Human Services (formerly Medicare Australia) enrolment database. Participants entered the study by completing a baseline postal questionnaire (between January 2006 and December 2009) and providing written consent to have their health followed over time. The sub-study surveys of women who indicated at the baseline that they had been diagnosed by a doctor as having osteoarthritis or osteoporosis, occurred between August and November 2016. A total of 640 women with osteoarthritis and 640 women with osteoporosis were mailed a questionnaire and of these women 404 (63.1 per cent) and 393 (61.4 per cent) returned completed sub-study questionnaires, respectively.

*Demographic characteristics*

Demographic measures included age, education (no formal schooling/school only, trade/apprentice/diploma, university degree), marital status (single, married/de facto, separated/divorced/widowed). Area of residence was defined using the ARIA+ remoteness score, which uses post code to determine road distances to service centres, and thus women were categorised as residing in a major city, inner regional area, or outer regional/remote area (AIHW, 2004). In addition, as a measure of income, women were asked how they managed on their available income ('it is impossible', 'it is difficult all the time', 'it is difficult some of the time', 'it is not too bad', 'it is easy').

*Self-care health practices or products*

The women were asked if they had used a range of self-care health practices or products specifically for their chronic illness in the previous 12 months. The practices or products included aromatherapy oils, herbal medicines, homeopathic remedies, multivitamins, meditation by themselves (i.e. without an instructor), yoga by themselves (i.e. without an instructor), and/or physical activities/exercise. If a woman indicated taking/using one or more of the self-care health practices or products, she was asked to indicate whether this use was effective (i.e. effective, somewhat effective, not at all effective).

*Statistical analyses*

A chi-square test, or Fisher's Exact test where appropriate, was used to examine the association between two categorical variables. Statistical significance was set at $p < 0.05$. All statistical analyses were undertaken using Stata 14.1.

## Results

The average age of the women was 71.3 (SD = 8.8) years, ranging from 53–94 years. The majority of the women resided in a major city (52.3 per cent), with 36.3 per cent residing in an inner regional area and 11.4 per cent in an outer regional area. Most of the women were married or in a de facto relationship (60.4 per cent), while 33.5 per cent were separated, divorced or widowed and 6.1 per cent were single. A university degree was attained by 30.1 per cent of the women, with 29.8 per cent completing a trade/apprenticeship or diploma, and 40.1 per cent having no formal education or attended school only. In terms of their ability to manage on available income, 71.0 per cent of the women indicated that they had little or no difficulties, 20.4 per cent indicated that they had some difficulties, and 8.6 per cent indicated that it was difficult or impossible all of the time.

The use of self-care health practices or products for osteoarthritis or osteoporosis is presented in Table 6.1. Overall, 55 per cent of the women used some form of complementary practices/products for their chronic illness; women with

*Table 6.1* The use of self-care products or practices for the treatment of osteoarthritis and osteoporosis symptoms

| Self-care products or practices | | Osteo-arthritis (n = 404) (%) | Osteo-porosis (n = 393) (%) | Total (n = 797) (%) | p-value |
|---|---|---|---|---|---|
| Aromatherapy oils | Yes | 7 | 3 | 5 | 0.005 |
| | No | 93 | 97 | 95 | |
| Herbal medicine | Yes | 8 | 4 | 6 | 0.031 |
| | No | 92 | 96 | 94 | |
| Homeopathic remedies | Yes | 2 | 1 | 1 | 0.546 |
| | No | 98 | 99 | 99 | |
| Multivitamins | Yes | 23 | 22 | 22 | 0.637 |
| | No | 77 | 78 | 78 | |
| Meditation | Yes | 11 | 8 | 10 | 0.233 |
| | No | 89 | 92 | 90 | |
| Yoga | Yes | 4 | 7 | 5 | 0.093 |
| | No | 96 | 93 | 95 | |
| Physical activity/ exercise | Yes | 42 | 42 | 42 | 0.922 |
| | No | 58 | 58 | 58 | |
| Total | Yes | 56 | 54 | 55 | 0.523 |
| | No | 44 | 46 | 45 | |

osteoarthritis being the highest users of self-care practices or products (56 per cent), followed by women with osteoporosis (54 per cent). Overall, the most popular self-care practices or products were physical activity/exercises (42 per cent), multivitamins (22 per cent), and meditation (10 per cent). In terms of differences between the osteoarthritis and osteoporosis groups, women with osteoarthritis were statistically significantly higher users of aromatherapy oils ($p = 0.005$) and/or herbal medicine ($p = 0.031$), compared to women with osteoporosis. There were no statistically significant differences between women with osteoarthritis or osteoporosis and use of any other self-care practices or products.

Table 6.2 shows the self-rated effectiveness of self-care health practices or products for relieving symptoms associated with osteoarthritis or osteoporosis. All of the self-care health practices and products, with the exception of homeopathy, were considered to effective or somewhat effective by most of the women (ranging from 76–99 per cent) who used them to relieve symptoms associated with either osteoarthritis or osteoporosis. For homeopathy, 57 per cent of women with osteoarthritis and 50 per cent of the women with osteoporosis who used homeopathic remedies, considered them effective. There was a statistically significant difference in the self-rated effectiveness of multivitamins between women with osteoarthritis and women with osteoporosis, where 87 per cent of women with osteoporosis rated multivitamins effective, compared to 76 per cent of women with osteoarthritis ($p = 0.001$).

*Table 6.2* The effectiveness of self-care products or practices for relieving symptoms associated with osteoarthritis and osteoporosis

| Self-care products or practices | | Osteo-arthritis (%) | Osteo-porosis (%) | p-value |
|---|---|---|---|---|
| Aromatherapy oils | Effective | 41 | 31 | 0.681 |
| | Somewhat effective | 45 | 46 | |
| | Not at all effective | 14 | 23 | |
| Herbal medicine | Effective | 21 | 47 | 0.215 |
| | Somewhat effective | 61 | 42 | |
| | Not at all effective | 18 | 11 | |
| Homeopathic remedies | Effective | 14 | 17 | 0.940 |
| | Somewhat effective | 43 | 33 | |
| | Not at all effective | 43 | 50 | |
| Multivitamins | Effective | 22 | 49 | 0.001 |
| | Somewhat effective | 54 | 38 | |
| | Not at all effective | 24 | 13 | |
| Meditation | Effective | 40 | 63 | 0.144 |
| | Somewhat effective | 47 | 37 | |
| | Not at all effective | 13 | 0 | |
| Yoga | Effective | 37 | 59 | 0.283 |
| | Somewhat effective | 53 | 41 | |
| | Not at all effective | 10 | 0 | |
| Physical activity/ exercise | Effective | 59 | 69 | 0.313 |
| | Somewhat effective | 39 | 30 | |
| | Not at all effective | 2 | 1 | |

## Discussion

Our analyses reveals a number of insights regarding CIM self-care use for osteoarthritis and osteoporosis. First, the prevalence of self-care practices/products among women with osteoarthritis and osteoporosis is high (55 per cent) particularly for physical activity/exercise (42 per cent), multivitamins (22 per cent), and meditation (10 per cent). Moreover, the pattern of use of self-care practices/products is similar across the two chronic illness for most of the self-care practices/products with two exceptions being higher prevalence of aromatherapy oils and herbal medicine use osteoarthritis for both groups of women.

Contrary to women diagnosed with osteoporosis, those diagnosed with osteoarthritis regularly experience joint pain and stiffness. A variety of herbal therapies have been used traditionally for the treatment of pain and potential inflammation, including arnica, boswellia, devil's claw and ginger. While oral and topical herbal therapies have regularly been promoted and used for osteoarthritis, the evidence is still inconclusive for most of those herbal preparations (Cameron & Chrubasik, 2014). For osteoporosis, on the other hand, no herbal therapies have been established, with some exceptions from Traditional Chinese Medicine herbal preparations (Leung & Siu, 2013). Similarly, aromatherapy may be beneficial for pain control in osteoarthritis with studies indicating significant pain reduction after the use of aromatherapy. Nevertheless, relevant studies have employed different essential oils, and partially applied aromatherapy in combination with heat, and/or massages, potentially boosting its efficacy.

Most of the women considered all (except homeopathy) self-care practices/ products to be effective or at least somewhat effective (ranging from 76–99 per cent). There was general agreement about the effectiveness of the self-care practices/products across the osteoarthritis and osteoporosis groups with the exception that the women reporting osteoporosis considered multivitamins to be more effective than those with osteoarthritis. Practices (exercise, meditation, yoga) were considered slightly more effective than products among both groups of women.

## Conclusion

As this chapter has shown, reframing certain CIM consumption as self-care behaviours and practices provides an excellent opportunity to gain insights into the role and consequence of CIM use for supporting women with chronic illness. Nevertheless, further research is needed to explore and help address a number of challenges to women achieving optimal relief from symptoms and a status of positive health. Given the potential direct and indirect risks of CIM self-care which are exacerbated by the lack of communication and non-disclosure, it is important that all providers (both CIM and conventionally located) consider and seek to engage women regarding these activities with a view to helping facilitate optimal care that incorporates or at least considers all health-seeking options women may undertake for their chronic illness.

## Acknowledgements

We are grateful to the women from the 45 and Up Study who consented to participate in our sub-study. We also thank the Australian Research Council for supporting this work via an ARC Discovery Project (DP1094765) and for supporting Professor Jon Adams while writing this chapter via an ARC Professorial Future Fellowship (FT140100195).

## References

45 and Up Study Collaborators (2008) Cohort profile: the 45 and Up Study. *International Journal of Epidemiology*, 37: 941–947.

Adams, J. (2017) Complementary and integrative medicine asnd patient self-management of health. *Complementary Medicine Research*, 24: 205-206.

Adams, J., Kroll, T, & Broom, A. (2014) The significance of complementary and alternative medicine as self-care: Examining 'hidden' health-seeking behaviour for chronic illness in later life. *Advances in Integrative Medicine* 1(3): 103–104.

Adams, J., Sibbritt, D., Lui, C., Broom, A., & Wardle, J. (2013) Omega-3 fatty acid supplement use in the 45 and Up cohort study. *BMJ Open* 3:e002292.

AIHW (Australian Institute of Health and Welfare) (2004) *Rural, Regional and Remote Health: A Guide to Remoteness Classifications.* Canberra: Australian Institute of Health and Welfare.

AIHW (Australian Institute of Health and Welfare). (2017) *The Burden of Musculoskeletal Conditions in Australia: A Detailed Analysis of the Australian Burden of Disease Study 2011.* Australian Burden of Disease Study series no. 13. BOD 14. Canberra: AIHW.

Altman, R., Alarcon, G., Appelrouth, D., et al. (1991) The American College of Rheumatology criteria for the classification and reporting of osteoarthritis of the hip. *Arthritis & Rheumatology*, 34(5): 505–514.

Altman, R., Asch, E., Bloch, D., Bole, G. et al. (1986) Development of criteria for the classification and reporting of osteoarthritis. Classification of osteoarthritis of the knee. Diagnostic and Therapeutic Criteria Committee of the American Rheumatism Association. *Arthritis & Rheumatology*, 29(8): 1039–1049.

Armstrong, A.R., Thiébaut, S.P., Brown, L.J. & Nepal, B. (2011) Australian adults use complementary and alternative medicine in the treatment of chronic illness: a national study, *Australian and New Zealand Journal of Public Health*, 35(4): 384–390.

Aspin, C., Jowsey, T., Glasgow, N. et al. (2010) Health policy responses to rising rates of multi-morbid chronic illness in Australia and New Zealand, *Australian and New Zealand Journal of Public Health*, 34(4): 386–393.

Avenell, A., Mak, J. C., & O'Connell, D. (2014) Vitamin D and vitamin D analogues for preventing fractures in post-menopausal women and older men. *Cochrane Database of Systematic Reviews* (4), Cd000227. doi:10.1002/14651858.CD000227.pub4.

Beaglehole, R., Reddy, S. & Leeder, S. R. (2007) Poverty and human development: the global implications of cardiovascular disease, *American Heart Association*, 116: 1871–1873.

Bishop, F. L. & Yardley, L. (2004) Constructing agency in treatment decisions: negotiating responsibility in cancer, *Health*, 8(4): 465–482.

Blaxter, M. (1976) *The Meaning of Disability: A Sociological Study of Impairment*, London: Heinemann Educational Publishers.

Broom, A. (2009) 'I'd forgotten about me in all of this': Discourses of self-healing, positivity and vulnerability in cancer patients' experiences of complementary and alternative medicine, *Journal of Sociology*, 45(1): 71–87.

Broom, A., Kirby, E., Sibbritt, D., Adams, J. & Refshauge, K. (2012) Use of complementary and alternative medicine by mid-age women with back pain: a national cross-sectional survey. *BMC Complementary and Alternative Medicine* 12: 98.

Broom, A., Meurk, C., Adams, J. & Sibbritt, D. (2014) My health, my responsibility? Complementary medicine and self (health) care, *Journal of Sociology*, 50(4): 515–530.

Brosseau, L., Taki, J., Desjardins, B. et al. (2017) The Ottawa Panel clinical practice guidelines for the management of knee osteoarthritis. Part one: introduction, and mind-body exercise programs. *Clinical Rehabilitation*, 31(5): 582–595. doi:10.1177/0269215517691083.

Brosseau, L., Yonge, K. A., Robinson, V. et al. (2003) Thermotherapy for treatment of osteoarthritis. *Cochrane Database of Systematic Reviews*, (4), Cd004522. doi:10.1002/14651858.cd004522.

Bury, M. (1982) Chronic illness as biographical disruption, *Sociology of Health & Illness*, 4(2): 167–182.

Cameron, M. & Chrubasik, S. (2013) Topical herbal therapies for treating osteoarthritis. *Cochrane Database of Syst Rev*(5), Cd010538. doi:10.1002/14651858.cd010538

Cameron, M. & Chrubasik, S. (2014) Oral herbal therapies for treating osteoarthritis. *Cochrane Database of Systematic Reviews*, (5), Cd002947. doi:10.1002/14651858.CD 002947.pub2.

Charmaz, K. (1983) Loss of self: a fundamental form of suffering in the chronically ill. *Sociology of Health & Illness*, 5(2): 168–195.

Corbin, J. M. & Strauss, A. (1988) *Unending Work and Care: Managing Chronic Illness at Home*, San Francisco: Jossey-Bass.

Coulter, I. (2004) Integration and paradigm clash. In P. Tovey (ed.), *Mainstreaming of Complementary and Alternative Medicine: Studies in Social Context*, London: Routledge.

Cramer, H., Ostermann, T. & Dobos, G. (2017) Injuries and other adverse events associated with yoga practice: a systematic review of epidemiological studies. *Journal of Science and Medicine in Sport*. doi:10.1016/j.jsams.2017.08.026.

Eriksen, E. F., Diez-Perez, A. & Boonen, S. (2014) Update on long-term treatment with bisphosphonates for postmenopausal osteoporosis: a systematic review. *Bone*, 58: 126–135. doi:10.1016/j.bone.2013.09.023.

Essue, B., Kelly, P., Roberts, M., Leeder, S. & Jan, S. (2011) We can't afford my chronic illness! The out-of-pocket burden associated with managing chronic obstructive pulmonary disease in Western Sydney, Australia, *Journal of Health Services Research & Policy*, 16(4): 226–231.

Feldman, S., Byles, J., Mishra, G. & Powers, J. (2002) The health and social needs of recently widowed older women in Australia, *Australasian Journal on Ageing*, 21(3): 135–140.

French, H. P., Brennan, A., White, B. & Cusack, T. (2011) Manual therapy for osteoarthritis of the hip or knee: a systematic review. *Manual Therapy*, 16(2): 109–117.

Gillespie, L. D., Robertson, M. C., Gillespie, W. J. et al. (2012) Interventions for preventing falls in older people living in the community. *Cochrane Database of Systematic Reviews* (9), Cd007146. doi:10.1002/14651858.CD007146.pub3.

Greenhalgh, T. (2009) Chronic illness: beyond the expert patient, *BMJ*, 338(7695): 629–631.

Gregory, S. (2005) Living with chronic illness in the family setting, *Sociology of Health & Illness*, 27(3): 372–392.

Guccione, A. A., Felson, D. T., Anderson, J. J., et al. (1994) The effects of specific medical conditions on the functional limitations of elders in the Framingham Study. *American Journal of Public Health*, 84(3): 351–358.

Gunn, J.M., Ayton, D.R., Densley, K. et al. (2012) The association between chronic illness, multimorbidity and depressive symptoms in an Australian primary care cohort, *Social Psychiatry and Psychiatric Epidemiology*, 47(2): 175–184.

Harris, M.F., Williams, A.M., Dennis, S.M., Zwar, N.A. & Davies, G.P. (2008) Chronic disease self-management: implementation with and within Australian general practice, *Medical Journal of Australia*, 189(10): S17.

Harris, P. E., Cooper, K. L., Relton, C. & Thomas, K. J. (2012) Prevalence of complementary and alternative medicine (CAM) use by the general population: a systematic review and update, *International Journal of Clinical Practice*, 66(10): 924–939.

Hochberg, M. C., Altman, R. D., April, K. T. et al. (2012) American College of Rheumatology 2012 recommendations for the use of nonpharmacologic and pharmacologic therapies in osteoarthritis of the hand, hip, and knee. *Arthritis Care and Research*, 64(4): 465–474.

Howe, T. E., Shea, B., Dawson, L. J. et al. (2011) Exercise for preventing and treating osteoporosis in postmenopausal women. *Cochrane Database of Systematic Reviews* (7), Cd000333. doi:10.1002/14651858.CD000333.pub2.

Jan, S., Essue, B.M. & Leeder, S.R. (2012) Falling through the cracks: the hidden economic burden of chronic illness and disability on Australian households, *Medical Journal of Australia*, 196(1): 29–31.

Jeon, Y. H., Jowsey, T., Yen, L. et al. (2010) Achieving a balanced life in the face of chronic illness, *Australian Journal of Primary Health*, 16(1): 66–74.

Jowsey, T., Jeon, Y. H., Dugdale, P. et al. (2009) Challenges for co-morbid chronic illness care and policy in Australia: a qualitative study, *Australia and New Zealand Health Policy*, 6(1): 22.

Kanis, J. A., Melton, L. J., 3rd, Christiansen, C., Johnston, C. C., & Khaltaev, N. (1994) The diagnosis of osteoporosis. *Journal of Bone and Mineral Research*, 9(8): 1137–1141. doi:10.1002/jbmr.5650090802.

Kennedy, A., Rogers, A. & Bower, P. (2007) Support for self-care for patients with chronic disease, *BMJ*, 335(7627): 968.

Lauche, R., Langhorst, J., Dobos, G., & Cramer, H. (2013) A systematic review and meta-analysis of Tai Chi for osteoarthritis of the knee. *Complementary Therapies in Medicine*, 21(4): 396-406. doi:10.1016/j.ctim.2013.06.001.

LeBoff, M. S., Kohlmeier, L., Hurwitz, S. et al. (1999) Occult vitamin D deficiency in postmenopausal US women with acute hip fracture. *JAMA*, 281(16): 1505–1511.

Leung, P. & Siu, W. (2013) Herbal treatment for osteoporosis: a current review. *Journal of Traditional and Complementary Medicine*, 3(2): 82–87.

Manheimer, E., Cheng, K., Linde, K. et al. (2010) Acupuncture for peripheral joint osteoarthritis. *Cochrane Database of Systematic Reviews*, (1), Cd001977. doi:10.1002/1465 1858.CD001977.pub2.

Nikander, R., Sievanen, H., Heinonen, A. et al. (2010) Targeted exercise against osteoporosis: a systematic review and meta-analysis for optimising bone strength throughout life. *BMC Medicine*, 8, 47. doi:10.1186/1741-7015-8-47.

Nissen, N. (2011) Challenging perspectives: women, complementary and alternative medicine, and social change, *Interface: A Journal for and about Social Movement*, 3: 187–212.

O'Neill, E.S. & Morrow, L.L. (2001) The symptom experience of women with chronic illness, *Journal of Advanced Nursing*, 33(2): 257–268.

Poole, K. E., & Compston, J. E. (2012) Bisphosphonates in the treatment of osteoporosis. *BMJ*, 344, e3211. doi:10.1136/bmj.e3211.

Rabenda, V., Hiligsmann, M. & Reginster, J. Y. (2009) Poor adherence to oral bisphosphonate treatment and its consequences: a review of the evidence. *Expert Opinion on Pharmacotherapy*, 10(14): 2303–2315. doi:10.1517/14656560903140533.

Reginster, J. Y. (2002) The prevalence and burden of arthritis. *Rheumatology (Oxford)*, 41(Suppl. 1), 3–6.

Reid, R., Steel, A., Wardle, J., Trubody, A. & Adams, J. (2016) Complementary medicine use by the Australian population: a critical mixed studies systematic review of utilisation, perceptions and factors associated with use, *BMC Complementary and Alternative Medicine*, 16: 176.

Sherrington, C., Whitney, J. C., Lord, S. R. et al. (2008) Effective exercise for the prevention of falls: a systematic review and meta-analysis. *Journal of the American Geriatric Society*, 56(12): 2234–2243. doi:10.1111/j.1532-5415.2008.02014.x.

Sibbritt, D., Adams, J., Lui, C.W., Broom, A. & Wardle, J. (2012) Who uses glucosamine and why? A study of 266,848 Australians aged 45 years and older, *PloS One*, 7(7): e41540.

Silverman, S. L., Schousboe, J. T. & Gold, D. T. (2011) Oral bisphosphonate compliance and persistence: a matter of choice? *Osteoporosis International*, 22(1), 21–26. doi:10.1007/s00198-010-1274-6.

Singh, J. A., Noorbaloochi, S., MacDonald, R. & Maxwell, L. J. (2015) Chondroitin for osteoarthritis. *Cochrane Database of Systematic Reviews*, 1, Cd005614. doi:10.1002/14651858.CD005614.pub2.

Sointu, E. (2006) Healing bodies, feeling bodies: embodiment and alternative and complementary health practices, *Social Theory & Health*, 4(3): 203–220.

The Royal Australian College of General Practitioners, & Osteoporosis Australia. (2017) *Osteoporosis Prevention, Diagnosis and Management in Postmenopausal Women and Men Over 50 Years of Age.* East Melbourne, VIC: RACGP.

Thorne, S., McCormick, J. & Carty, E. (1997) Deconstructing the gender neutrality of chronic illness and disability, *Health Care for Women International*, 18(1): 1–16.

Towheed, T. E., Maxwell, L., Anastassiades, T. P. et al. (2005) Glucosamine therapy for treating osteoarthritis. *Cochrane Database of Systematic Reviews* (2), Cd002946. doi:10.1002/14651858.CD002946.pub2.

Townsend, A., Wyke, S. & Hunt, K. (2006) Self-managing and managing self: practical and moral dilemmas in accounts of living with chronic illness, *Chronic Illness*, 2(3): 185–194.

Tsai, P. F., Chang, J. Y., Beck, C., Hagen, J. et al. (2009) The feasibility of implementing Tai Chi for nursing home residents with knee osteoarthritis and cognitive impairment. *Activities Directors' Quarterly for Alzheimers and Other Dement Patients*, 10(1): 9–17.

Walker, C. (2010) Ruptured identities: leaving work because of chronic illness, *International Journal of Health Services*, 40(4): 629–643.

Wang, C., Schmid, C. H., Iversen, M. D. et al. (2016) Comparative effectiveness of Tai Chi versus physical therapy for knee osteoarthritis: a randomized trial. *Annals of International Medicine*, 165(2): 77–86. doi:10.7326/m15-2143.

Watts, J. J., Abimanyi-Ochom, J. & Sanders, K. M. (2013) *Osteoporosis Costing All Australian: A New Burden of Disease Analysis – 2012 to 2022.* Melbourne, VIC: Osteoporosis Australia.

Wayne, P. M., Berkowitz, D. L., Litrownik, D. E., Buring, J. E. & Yeh, G. Y. (2014) What do we really know about the safety of Tai Chi?: A systematic review of adverse event reports in randomized trials. *Archives of Physical Medicine and Rehabilitation*, 95(12): 2470–2483. doi:10.1016/j.apmr.2014.05.005,

Wayne, P. M., Kiel, D. P., Krebs, D. E. et al. (2007) The effects of Tai Chi on bone mineral density in postmenopausal women: a systematic review. *Archives of Physical Medicine and Rehabilitation*, 88(5): 673–680. doi:10.1016/j.apmr.2007.02.012.

Wellard, S. (2010) Globalisation of chronic illness research, in D. Kralik, B. Paterson & V. Coates (eds) *Translating Chronic Illness Research into Practice*, Oxford: Blackwell.

Werner, A., Isaksen, L.W. & Malterud, K. (2004) 'I am not the kind of woman who complains of everything': illness stories on self and shame in women with chronic pain, *Social Science & Medicine*, 59(5): 1035–1045.

WHO (World Health Organization). (1994) Assessment of fracture risk and its application to screening for postmenopausal osteoporosis: report of a WHO study group meeting held in Rome, 22–25 June 1992.

WHO (World Health Organization). (2009) *Self-care in the Context of Primary Health Care*, Bangkok, Thailand: World Health Organization.

WHO (World Health Organization). (2017) Noncommunicable diseases. Fact Sheet. Available at: www.cdc.gov/chronicdisease/overview/index.htm (accessed 20 December 2017).

Wilson, S. (2007) 'When you have children, you're obliged to live': motherhood, chronic illness and biographical disruption, *Sociology of Health & Illness*, 29(4): 610–626.

Xue, C.C., Zhang, A.L., Da Costa, C. & Story, D.F. (2007) Complementary and alternative medicine use in Australia: a national population-based survey, *The Journal of Alternative and Complementary Medicine*, 13(6): 643–650.

Yang, L., Sibbritt, D. & Adams, J. (2017) A critical review of complementary and alternative medicine use among people with arthritis: a focus upon prevalence, cost, user profiles, motivation, decision-making, perceived benefits and communication. *Rheumatology International*, *37*(3), 337–351. doi:10.1007/s00296-016-3616-y.

# 7   Women's mental health and complementary and integrative medicine

*Erica McIntyre, Jane Frawley and Romy Lauche*

## Introduction

Mental health disorders are highly prevalent, with women being more likely than men to experience either a mood or anxiety disorder. The aim of this chapter is to explore complementary and integrative medicine (CIM) use for the two most prevalent mental health conditions: depression and anxiety. We begin this chapter by outlining the worldwide prevalence of depression and anxiety, and present a brief review of these common mental health disorders. We also describe CIM use by women for the treatment of depression and anxiety, and the evidence base for the most commonly used CIM for these conditions. The model of integrative mental health care (IMHC) is explored and, we argue, is an important model for providing optimal mental health outcomes for women. Finally, we discuss the barriers to facilitating IMHC and identify research objectives for achieving quality IMHC for women.

## Prevalence of mental health disorders

Depression and anxiety are common illnesses worldwide, with more than 300 million people (4.4 per cent of the total global population) affected by depression and 260 million people (3.6 per cent of the total global population) affected by an anxiety disorder (World Health Organization 2017). The burden of disease from mental health conditions is on the rise globally, with a 4.4 per cent increase in the global prevalence of depression, and a 3.6 per cent increase in the global prevalence of anxiety from 2005 to 2015 (ibid.). Together, depression and anxiety disorders cost the global economy US$1 trillion each year (World Health Organization 2016).

Depression can be defined as depressed mood or loss of interest and pleasure, with at least four additional symptoms present for two or more weeks:

- significant weight change;
- insomnia or hypersomnia;
- psychomotor agitation or retardation;
- fatigue;

- feelings of worthlessness or excessive guilt;
- poor concentration;
- recurrent thoughts of death, including fear of dying;
- suicidal ideation or a suicide attempt.

Generalised anxiety disorder may be diagnosed when excessive anxiety and worry about various events or activities occur more days than not for at least 6 months. In adults, anxiety and worry are associated with at least three of the following symptoms (restlessness, fatigue, difficulty concentrating, irritability, muscle tension, poor sleep). Panic disorder, specific phobias, post-traumatic stress disorder, and obsessive-compulsive disorder exhibit variations of anxiety symptoms. For a depression or anxiety disorder diagnosis, symptoms of depression and anxiety must cause clinically significant distress or impair functioning and not be attributed to substance abuse or be caused by another medical disorder.

A systematic review and meta-analysis of 174 studies conducted in a variety of high-, low-, and middle-income countries found one in five adults (17.6 per cent) had experienced a common mental disorder in the previous 12 months, with nearly one-third of adults (29.2 per cent) experiencing a mental health problem in their lifetime (Steel et al. 2014). In total, mental disorders account for 30 per cent of the global non-fatal disease burden (World Health Organization 2017). A review of 87 studies from 44 countries found a current prevalence of anxiety disorders (adjusted for methodological differences) at 7.3 per cent (4.8–10.9 per cent). European/Anglo cultures report a higher overall prevalence of 10.4 per cent (7.0–15.5 per cent) compared to 5.3 per cent (3.5–8.1 per cent), for African cultures (Baxter et al. 2013). The large variability in prevalence estimates was due to a range of factors such as culture, age, area of residence (urban or rural), economic status, and gender.

Women are more likely to experience depression or anxiety disorder compared to men (Steel et al. 2014), and between 2.6 per cent and 43.9 per cent of women have been found to suffer from depression, with younger women and specific population groups reporting higher prevalence rates (Rich et al. 2013). Previous mental health disorders, increasing age, smoking, adverse life events, and being a single parent are all associated with the increased likelihood of developing depression (ibid.).

Mental health disorders such as depression and anxiety lead to substantial personal losses in health and functioning as well as wider family, societal and economic costs (World Health Organization 2016). Such personal and societal burdens can be measured at the population level by multiplying the average level of disability associated with these conditions by the proportion of the global population living with mental health disorders. This formula estimates the Years Lived with Disability (YLD). In 2015, it was estimated that depressive disorders were responsible for over 50 million YLD and anxiety was associated with 24.6 million YLD (World Health Organization 2017). Depression is the largest contributor to non-fatal health loss globally, with anxiety as the sixth largest contributor (ibid.). The majority of this non-fatal disease burden occurred in low-income and middle-income countries.

## CIM: an important treatment option for women with mental health problems

There are a number of evidence-based conventional medical treatments available to women who experience anxiety or depression, which include psychological and pharmacological therapies (McIntyre et al. 2014). In many cases, these treatments are critical for the management of anxiety or depressive disorders. However, there are also many people who do not benefit from these treatments, such as those with subthreshold symptoms (Barbui et al. 2011). A range of issues have been associated with the use of pharmaceuticals for the treatment of anxiety and depression including: a lack of response to treatment and relapse, unwanted side-effects, risk of dependency, and lack of suitability for long-term treatment (Pigott et al. 2010). There are also unique issues for women – for example, for pregnant women, there is increased risk of spontaneous abortion for certain classes of antidepressants (Nakhai-Pour et al. 2010), and an increased risk of children developing risk of attention-deficit/hyperactivity disorder with the use of bupropion during pregnancy (Figueroa 2010). Psychological therapies are also not always suitable, with a lack of access to practitioner-led therapies related to cost and physical barriers, and lack of response to psychological therapies and relapse. The non-response rates for conventional treatments have been estimated at more than 30 per cent for anxiety (Taylor et al. 2012), and over 50 per cent for depression (Wiles et al. 2014). Consequently, other treatment options are needed to address these treatment gaps and suit individual needs.

Treatment effects also vary according to gender, as women are biologically and psychologically different to men. These differences can affect the pharmacokinetics of certain pharmaceuticals, with differences in metabolism, efficacy, and side-effects (Sramek and Cutler 2011). For example, women tend to experience a greater severity of anxiety symptoms compared to men and are thereby more likely to be non-responders to both cognitive-behaviour therapy and pharmaceutical treatments (Taylor et al. 2012). In addition, women have specific health needs, hormonal differences, and certain life stages (e.g. pregnancy and menopause) that require consideration by health practitioners when treating mental health problems.

CIM is a popular treatment choice for mental health problems (McIntyre et al. 2015; Solomon and Adams 2015; Reid et al. 2016). However, the current prevalence of CIM use by women for various CIM mental health conditions is unknown. Having a mental health disorder has been found to predict the use of CIM (McIntyre et al. 2016). The 2007 National Mental Health Survey in Australia reported over 70 per cent of CIM users as having a mental health condition, and that having a mental disorder diagnosis predicted CIM use (Spinks and Hollingsworth 2012). A review of international studies has found that between 10 and 30 per cent of people experiencing depressive disorders use some form of CIM, and that depressive symptoms occur with greater prevalence in CIM users compared to non-users (Solomon and Adams 2015). In addition, severity of symptoms has been associated with CIM use, for example, anxiety symptoms have been found to predict herbal medicine use (McIntyre et al. 2017).

Various clinical guidelines now incorporate the need to consider CIM as a treatment option for mental health problems (Malhi et al. 2015). Recommended strategies include the adoption of evidence-based CIM by conventional practitioners, and consultation with CIM practitioners into mainstream health care systems if appropriate, with consideration of women's treatment preferences related to their individual needs and personal values. For example, St John's wort has demonstrated efficacy in the treatment of mild to moderate depression equal to that of first-line antidepressant medications (Maher et al. 2016), has fewer side-effects than pharmaceutical treatments, and is a more cost-effective treatment compared to conventional anti-depressants (Solomon et al. 2013). As such, it is likely that many women could benefit from the use of St John's wort and other evidence-based CIM to assist in managing mental health conditions.

## Evidence-based complementary medicine for common mental health disorders

While evidence for the efficacy of most CIM interventions is still sparse, existing studies suggest that certain interventions might be effective, and safe for specific mental health problems. The types of CIM discussed below include mind-body medicines (e.g., meditation or yoga), biological medicines (e.g., herbs or nutritionals), and whole systems of care (e.g., naturopathy or traditional Chinese medicine).

### Mind-body medicine

Mind-body medicine is an umbrella term covering a wide variety of therapeutic techniques focusing on the ways in which emotional, mental, social, spiritual, experiential, and behavioural factors can directly affect health. The main techniques include mindfulness interventions (in the form of mindfulness-based cognitive therapy or mindfulness-based stress reduction) and meditation, but also exercise interventions such as yoga, Tai Chi or qigong, and relaxation training. While these techniques do not provide a cure for depression or anxiety, they may improve mental health symptoms and general well-being (D'Silva et al. 2012).

### Mindfulness interventions

Mindfulness interventions include a group of treatments derived from traditional meditation and yoga techniques. Mindfulness-based cognitive therapy (MBCT), a combination of cognitive therapy with mindfulness elements, has been developed for the management of depressive disorders, with one systematic review indicating that it might prevent depressive relapse in individuals with recurring depression (Fjorback et al. 2011).

Mindfulness-based stress reduction (MBSR) – an 8-week standardised programme using mindfulness meditation, body awareness training, and yoga – has also been shown to improve mental health outcomes in both healthy participants and clinical populations with psychiatric disorders (ibid.). For meditation – 'a family of self-regulation practices that focus[es] on training attention and awareness in order to bring mental processes under greater voluntary control' (Walsh and Shapiro 2006) – small to moderate effects have been found in reducing depression and anxiety symptoms (Goyal et al. 2014). One systematic review and meta-analysis (n = 39 studies) of mindfulness-based treatments (MBCT and MBSR) identified large effects for both anxiety and depression symptoms (Hofmann et al. 2010).

Another form of cognitive therapy, acceptance and commitment therapy (ACT), which incorporates acceptance and mindfulness strategies, has also been found to be effective for depression. Evidence for anxiety disorders is still limited due to paucity of studies (Powers et al. 2009). However, one randomised controlled trial (RCT) (n = 128) comparing the efficacy of ACT to cognitive behavioural therapy (CBT) – a gold standard psychological treatment – for anxiety disorders (mixed) found that ACT was more effective in reducing anxiety disorder severity (Arch et al. 2012). The study also found a significant improvement in quality of life for the ACT treatment. However, CBT showed greater improvement compared to ACT.

### Exercise interventions

One of the most common recommendations for health and well-being is to remain physically activity, and to exercise regularly. Physical exercises may not only improve physical health, but can also prevent and reduce depressive symptoms, and the effects of exercise are mostly comparable to psychological interventions or drug therapy (Cooney et al. 2013). Exercise has also been found to improve anxiety disorder symptoms when employed complementary to conventional treatment (Jayakody et al. 2014).

Yoga is a group of traditional Indian physical, mental, and spiritual practices that originated around 5,000 years ago (Iyengar 1965). Modern yoga forms are frequently associated with physical postures, breathing techniques, and meditation. One recent systematic review found yoga as effective as medication and other forms of exercise for depressive symptoms (Cramer et al. 2017). Another review found yoga effective in reducing anxiety in individuals with elevated levels of anxiety even though it was not effective for individuals with manifest anxiety disorders (Cramer, in press). However, there are far fewer studies available for yoga and treatment of anxiety than for yoga and depression. Similar positive effects on depression and anxiety have been found in Tai Chi and qigong trials, despite there being fewer studies in general (Wang et al. 2014).

## Relaxation interventions

Relaxation techniques such as progressive muscle relaxation, relaxation imagery, or autogenic training might constitute psychological treatments for depression not requiring extensive training or costs. While studies suggest these techniques may not be as effective as psychological therapies like CBT, relaxation interventions could be considered potential psychological interventions for depression (Jorm et al. 2008).

## Herbal medicines

Herbal medicines have been used since antiquity for anxiety and depression symptoms, and a variety of herbs are available for these conditions with varying levels of efficacy (Sarris et al. 2013). While many of these medicines demonstrate promising results in clinical trials for specific presentations of depression and anxiety, for the majority, more research is needed to establish efficacy and long-term safety.

The most commonly used herbal medicine for depression is St. John's wort (*Hypericum perforatum*), which has good evidence of efficacy for mild to moderate depression compared to placebo in patients with major depressive disorder and is similarly effective while having fewer side effects than standard antidepressants (Maher et al. 2016). Other herbal medicines with emerging clinical evidence for treating depression symptoms include saffron (*Crocus sativus*) (Lopresti and Drummond 2014), turmeric (*Curcumin longa*) (Ng et al. 2017), red feather (*Echium amoenum*), lavender (*Lavendula angustifolia*) (Akhondzadeh et al. 2003) and the herb *Rhodiola rosea* (Hung et al. 2011).

The herb kava (*Piper methysticum*) has demonstrated strong evidence for the treatment of generalised anxiety (Camfield et al. 2017). However, there have been concerns about potential hepatotoxicity, which resulted in the withdrawal of kava products from Australian and European markets in 2002 (Sarris and McIntyre 2017). More recently these concerns have been addressed, with ethanolic preparations identified as the likely cause of hepatotoxic effects; consequently, aqueous preparations are recommended, and have been reintroduced to the Australian market (Sarris et al. 2011). Other herbal medicines with clinical trial evidence for reducing anxiety symptoms include ginkgo (*Gingko biloba*), lavender (*Lavandula angustifolia*), valerian (*Valeriana officinalis*), German chamomile (*Matricaria recutita*), lemon balm (*Melissa officinalis*), and passionflower (*Passiflora incarnata*). However, more research is needed on the effects of specific herbs in specific presentations of anxiety (Camfield et al. 2017).

## Nutritional medicine

It is now well recognised that nutrition plays a key role in mental health. Consuming traditional diets, such as the Mediterranean diet, is associated with the prevention of depression (Rienks et al. 2012), and an improvement in depression symptoms

100    *E. McIntyre, J. Frawley, R. Lauche*

(Opie et al. 2015). Nutritional medicines have also become a popular treatment for depression symptoms. A recent systematic review and meta-analysis of adjunctive (complementary) nutritional treatments for depression concluded that methylfolate, S-adenosyl-methionine (SAMe), omega-3 fatty acids (specifically eicosapentaenoic acid (EPA) or ethyl EPA), and vitamin D each significantly reduce depression symptoms to varying degrees (Sarris et al. 2016). Of note, EPA-rich omega-3 fish oil showed a significant reduction in depression symptoms compared to placebo, and can safely be used as an adjunctive treatment. It is worth noting that the majority of participants in the studies reviewed were female; consequently, these nutritional medicines are important considerations for women with depression symptoms.

Evidence for nutritional medicines in treating anxiety symptoms is emerging. The majority of clinical trials to date suggest magnesium, multivitamins (including B vitamins), L-lysine and L-arginine can reduce stress or anxiety to varying degrees (Camfield et al. 2017). However, as there are only a small number of studies of varying quality, more research is needed.

*Acupuncture*

Evidence for the efficacy of acupuncture for mental health is very limited, and considered insufficient for depression (Smith et al. 2010). As such, it cannot be recommended for the treatment of depression and anxiety at this stage.

*CIM systems: naturopathy*

Complementary medical systems such as traditional Chinese medicine, Ayurveda, Western herbal medicine, and naturopathy incorporate unique philosophies and treatments. There are few studies that explore the effectiveness of these medical systems for mental health conditions. Two studies have explored the effectiveness of naturopathic medicine – a holistic approach to managing health based on the principle that the body has the inherent ability to heal itself, with an emphasis on the use of natural treatments, such as nutritional and herbal medicines – for anxiety or depression. Naturopathy does not focus treatment on the depression in isolation, but takes a biopsychosocial approach that addresses general health status, health behaviours, and environment, and aims to treat the individual holistically to both prevent and treat mental health problems in addition to improving general well-being (Sarris et al. 2014a).

An Australian study (n = 11) suggests clinically significant improvements in self-reported anxiety, depression and stress symptoms for usual naturopathic treatment. However, the sample was too small to draw strong conclusions (Sarris et al. 2014a). Another study, a RCT (n = 75) of Canadian adults with self-reported anxiety, found that standardised naturopathic treatment significantly reduced anxiety symptoms to a greater extent than standard psychological therapy (counselling plus cognitive behavioural therapy) (Cooley et al. 2009). These studies provide preliminary evidence for the benefits of naturopathic treatment for common mental health problems.

## IMHC: the way forward

As discussed, conventional medicines are not necessarily suitable for all women. Consequently, it is essential that evidence-based CIM (treatments and medical systems) are appropriately integrated into mainstream health care. IMHC aims to facilitate a more inclusive, holistic approach that emphasises the importance of prevention and wellness (Sarris et al. 2014b). This approach is a reaction to the complex nature of mental health disorders, and the lack of improvement in treatment outcomes with conventional therapies. Sarris and colleagues (ibid.) propose a model of integrative mental health incorporating the use of CIM with the aim of addressing the challenges of conventional medical treatments, such as poor adherence, lack of access to mental health services, inadequate treatment effectiveness, and side effects of pharmaceuticals.

Monotherapy (use of only one treatment type, such as an antidepressant) is not considered suitable for treating mental health disorders, which is reflected in current treatment guidelines; for example, see the National Institute for Health and Care Excellence (2009). Treating mental health disorders is complex, involving multifactorial aetiology regarding physiological, psychological, social, and environmental factors. Consequently, recovery from mental health problems requires a holistic biopsychosocial approach considering all these factors, which is best achieved with a team-based approach to mental health care that acknowledges each person's treatment preferences (Department of Health and Ageing 2013). IMHC aims to incorporate the best of both conventional and CIM (including self-care) and health services, to optimise safe and effective treatment outcomes.

The pluralistic attitudes advocating exclusive use of one medical paradigm over the other within both conventional medicine and CIM has frequently been criticised, with consistent calls for integration (Hawk et al. 2015; Sarris et al. 2014b). Given the widespread use of CIM for mental health problems the integration of these treatments and services into mainstream healthcare needs urgent consideration by policy-makers and health practitioners. Integration of evidence-based CIM and health services will better enable people with mental health disorders to receive safe and effective treatments (Sarris et al. 2014b).

The holistic philosophies of CIM systems (e.g., naturopathy) make them well suited to play an important role in the management of mental health, and may assist in easing the burden on health care systems. It is estimated that only 46 per cent of people with a mental health problem received treatment from 2009–2010 (Whiteford et al. 2014), and providing improved access to *all* relevant mental health practitioners is a critical consideration requiring CIM practitioners to have adequate training in mental health.

The White Paper by Sarris and colleagues (2014b) recommends facilitating increased awareness of evidence-based CIM. As discussed previously, there is a growing evidence base for CIM and these have the potential to assist in preventing more severe anxiety and mood disorders, and improve depression and anxiety symptoms. Meanwhile, critics of CIM suggest that only the highest level of evidence (i.e., gold standard RCTs) can lead to mainstream acceptance, but this approach would exclude many treatments currently used in mainstream health care (Grossman and Mackenzie 2005), and the use of evidence-based practice incorporating all levels of evidence, including traditional evidence when appropriate, is needed (Leach 2016).

It is also important to recognise the treatment preferences of women. Women have been found to be significantly more likely to choose psychological therapy over pharmacotherapy (McHugh et al. 2013), and, as discussed previously, are high users of CIM. Therefore, the attitudes and beliefs of women need to be respected and considered when engaging in shared decision-making about mental health care. Effective integration also relies on ensuring women and health practitioners have access to accurate and reliable information on CIM for treating mental health problems; consequently, it is in the best interest of the public that an appropriate level of CIM education is incorporated into mainstream mental health care.

## Barriers to facilitating IMHC

Poor rates of disclosure of CIM use have been reported for pregnant women (Frawley et al., 2013; Frawley et al. 2016) and women with back pain (Murthy et al. 2017) leading to concerns about potential side effects, drug interactions and ineffective treatment and there is evidence this may also be a challenge regarding women with mental health disorders. A recent study of 400 adults with anxiety found that only half of the respondents reported disclosing their use of herbal medicine to their general practitioner (GP) (McIntyre et al. 2016).

### Shared decision making

Shared decision-making is considered best practice in mental health care (Department of Health and Ageing 2013). However, a complex set of circumstances make this challenging. CIM self-prescription is common among women with anxiety and depression (McIntyre et al. 2016). Research has also shown that women commonly rely on advice about CIM from family and friends and the Internet, and use CIM alongside prescription medicine for anxiety and depression, often without disclosing this use to health care providers (ibid.). Without disclosure of CIM use, the ability of medical providers to successfully manage safe CIM use is extremely challenging. However, general practitioners, psychologists and other mental health care providers may lack the necessary skills and knowledge to have effective conversations with women about CIM. Poor CIM literacy for GPs combined with time pressure may result in ineffective conversations. Research has found GPs feel inadequately equipped to discuss patients' CIM use (Pirotta et al. 2014), and are challenged in identifying good quality research on CIM (McGuire et al. 2009).

## Communication between conventional medical and CIM practitioners

Successful communication channels between conventional medical and CIM practitioners would facilitate patient-centred IMHC. A study of CIM practitioner (naturopaths, Western herbalists) referral practices for clients in their care with depression, anxiety or insomnia found 75 per cent had referred patients to mental health professionals (Morgan and Francis 2008). Approximately half of the naturopaths and herbalists had received referrals from conventional mental health practitioners. The lack of registration of CIM professions in many countries may act as a barrier to effective referral networks. Both regulation and registration differ from country to country and in many cases from state to state. For example, naturopaths are licensed as health practitioners in many parts in the United States but do not have the same regulation in the United Kingdom or Australia. Lack of CIM regulation may be inhibiting channels of communication between conventional medical practitioners and CIM practitioners.

## CIM practitioners' ability to manage mental health

There is also a need to understand how CIM practitioners treat and manage clients with mental health conditions in their care. While clinical guidelines exist for medical and allied health practitioners working in the area of mental health (e.g., general practitioners, psychologists, psychiatrists), no such guidelines exists for CIM practitioners who are frequently visited for mental health advice (Camfield et al. 2017). In addition, there is a lack of standardised training for many CIM practitioners, making it very difficult to even ascertain if CIM practitioners are adequately trained in mental health. A detailed understanding of the treatment frameworks and prescribing practices of a range of CIM practices is urgently needed.

## Cost of CIM health services

While some conventional health providers may recommend women in their care consult with a CIM practitioner, the cost of both practitioner visits and products may be prohibitive for many women. In Australia, the National Perinatal Depression Initiative was founded to encourage women in the perinatal period (pregnancy through to the end of the first postnatal year) to access mental health services under the Medicare Benefits Schedule if required (Chambers et al. 2016). An increased number of women have used the Medicare-funded mental health services after the introduction of this initiative (ibid.), and it is possible that the government subsidy encouraged women to seek help. Correspondingly, the high out-of-pocket cost of CIM practitioners and products may act as a barrier for women seeking care within the perinatal period and beyond. A recent study found that the average out-of-pocket spend by pregnant women accessing CIM practitioners was AU$185.40 and the average spend on CIM products was AU$179.60

(Adams et al. 2017). Further research from Australia has found that women with depression are more likely to self-prescribe CIM if they are not receiving conventional treatment (Adams et al. 2012), which may result from the high out-of-pocket spend to consult a CIM practitioner.

## Research objectives for achieving quality IMHC for women

While the evidence base for the efficacy of CIM interventions is growing, research gaps remain. In the following section a number of areas for future research are presented.

### *Workforce*

There is only limited published work of how CIM practitioners manage and treat people experiencing depression and anxiety, and an understanding of the actual practice of CIM practitioners with regards to mental health is urgently needed. For example, enquiry can determine who the practitioners are that treat mental health disorders, and what their training and qualifications are with regards to mental health. Studies need to determine how these providers are managing treatment (i.e., which tools they use for diagnosing, and monitoring), as well as the interventions and medicines they prescribe for the treatment of depression and anxiety, and whether these approaches are successful in improving mental health in people experiencing depression and anxiety.

### *Health practitioner communication*

Another important issue is the communication, including between health care practitioners, between patients and different health care providers, and the beliefs and attitudes that are reflected in the communication patterns. Patients often report dissatisfaction with the medical encounter regarding the use of CIM practices and products (McIntyre et al. 2015), and the lack of professional evidence-based communication can be considered a barrier for patients to find effective, coordinated and safe integrative health care. While integrative approaches to care within conventional medicine have emerged (Gureje et al. 2015), the dearth of research examining how medical doctors, mental health care providers and CIM providers can work together, and how collaboration can be strengthened has limited such integrative approaches. Specifically, no studies have been conducted to date to examine communication and referral patterns around mental illness and focus has been limited to communication and referral patterns among mental health specialists such as psychiatrists, psychologists and psychotherapists, a situation that urgently needs redress via future research.

### *Clinical research*

RCTs have long been considered the gold standard and the predominant source to generate evidence of the benefits of CIM interventions for depression and anxiety.

Such a design is often not applicable to the majority of people with depression and anxiety (Pigott et al. 2010), and more pragmatic or comparative effectiveness trials are needed to examine the benefits of CIM interventions in real-world clinical practice. For example, in women with different levels of depression and anxiety or potential comorbidities, or in comparison to established and effective treatments like specific types of psychotherapy. Trials also often do not include minorities, or disadvantaged populations who might have different needs and/or respond to the tested interventions in other ways (e.g., women compared to men).

Evidence from single intervention studies cannot be translated into the use of these treatments in combination with other treatments, or as part of whole medical systems. Traditional medicine systems often use a different approach to diagnosing physical and mental health conditions, which cannot compare to conventional medical diagnostic systems. Consequently, it is critical to consider an intervention's heritage, and traditional application as part of a whole medical system when designing clinical research.

### Health literacy

The current level of health literacy in the public can be considered low with regards to both mental health (Furnham and Lousley 2013) and CIM (Shreffler-Grant et al. 2013). While mental health literacy has improved over recent decades, there is still a lack of recognition of mental disorders, and a subset of negative beliefs and attitudes associated with mental illness (e.g., mental illness is a sign of weakness, interventions are not helpful) reducing help-seeking intentions and creating stigma (Clement et al. 2015). The lack of knowledge about CIM and communication on the part of conventional health care providers impacts on people with depression and anxiety with regards to their CIM use, leaving them unable to identify evidence-based information on CIM interventions from their primary health care providers. Many patients may thereby fail to explore effective CIM interventions or use CIM unsupervised, placing them at risk from ineffective, or even harmful advice and interventions (Wardle and Adams 2012). In order to improve health literacy among patients and providers, studies are necessary to determine the current status of mental health and CIM literacy, and to design interventions that might improve knowledge, access to evidence, and skills to navigate through the health care system and to facilitate informed, coordinated health care for the benefits of patients and public health.

### Health behaviour

While several factors such as age, gender and socio-economic status are well known to affect health behaviour, a substantial part of why and how people choose specific types of medicines and practitioners is still hidden. With steady increases in the use of non-professional information sources about CIM, an in-depth understanding is needed to examine why people are relying on such sources, and how that influences the ways they discuss the use of certain medicines and products with their health care providers. Future research also needs to take into account psychosocial and environmental factors when analysing driving forces of specific health behaviours, and identify ways to foster healthy lifestyle behaviours.

## Conclusion

This chapter has focused on depression and anxiety as experienced by women, and provided an overview of CIM use related to these conditions. Women are high users of CIM for mental health problems, as they are potentially filling a gap in treatment need, or CIM may align with their personal beliefs. However, due to a range of complex circumstances, women may not be using these medicines safely or effectively. Consequently, there is an urgent need for an integrative approach to the management of mental health to help mitigate the risks associated with inadequate diagnosis and treatment and ensure women are empowered to make adequately informed choices about their mental health care, including CIM use.

## References

Adams, J., Sibbritt, D., and Lui, C. (2012) Health service use among persons with self-reported depression: a longitudinal analysis of 7,164 women. *Archives of Psychiatric Nursing*, 26: 181–191.

Adams, J., Steel, A., Frawley, J. et al. (2017) Substantial out-of-pocket expenditure on maternity care practitioner consultations and treatments during pregnancy: estimates from a nationally-representative sample of pregnant women in Australia. *BMC Pregnancy Childbirth*, 17: 114.

Akhondzadeh, S., Kashani, L., Fotouhi, A. et al. (2003) Comparison of Lavandula angustifolia Mill. tincture and imipramine in the treatment of mild to moderate depression: a double-blind, randomized trial. *Progress in Neuro-Psychopharmacology and Biological Psychiatry*, 27: 123–127.

Arch, J., Eifert, G., Davies, C. et al. (2012) Randomized clinical trial of cognitive behavioral therapy (CBT) versus acceptance and commitment therapy (ACT) for mixed anxiety disorders. *Journal of Consulting and Clinical Psychology*, 80: 750–765.

Barbui, C., Cipriani, A., Patel, V. et al. (2011) Efficacy of antidepressants and benzo-diazepines in minor depression: systematic review and meta-analysis. *The British Journal of Psychiatry*, 198: 11–16.

Baxter, A. J., Scott, K. M., Vos, T. et al. (2013) Global prevalence of anxiety disorders: a systematic review and meta-regression. *Psychological Medicine*, 43: 897–910.

Camfield D. A., McIntyre, E. and Sarris, J. (2017) *Evidence-Based Herbal and Nutritional Treatment for Anxiety in Psychiatric Disorders*, Cham, Switzerland: Springer International Publishing.

Chambers, G. M., Randall, S., Hoang, V. P. et al. (2016) The National Perinatal Depression Initiative: an evaluation of access to general practitioners, psychologists and psychiatrists through the Medicare Benefits Schedule. *Australian and New Zealand Journal of Psychiatry*, 50: 264–274.

Clement, S., Schauman, O., Graham, T. et al. (2015) What is the impact of mental health-related stigma on help-seeking? A systematic review of quantitative and qualitative studies. *Psychological Medicine*, 45: 11–27.

Cooley, K., Szczurko, O., Perri, D. et al. (2009) Naturopathic care for anxiety: a randomized controlled trial ISRCTN78958974. *PLOS ONE*, 4: e6628.

Cooney, GM, Dwan, K, Greig, C. A. et al. (2013) Exercise for depression. *Cochrane Database of Systematic Reviews*, Cd004366.

Cramer, H., Anheyer, D., Lauche, R. et al. (2017) A systematic review of yoga for major depressive disorder. *Journal of Affective Disorders*, 213: 70–77.

Cramer, H., Lauche, R., Anheyer, D., Pilkington, K., de Manincor, M., Dobos G., and Ward, L. (in press) Yoga for anxiety: a systematic review and meta-analysis of randomized controlled trials. *Depression and Anxiety*.

Department of Health and Ageing. (2013) *National Framework for Recovery-Oriented Mental Health Services: Guide for Practitioners and Providers*, Canberra, ACT: Commonwealth of Australia.

D'Silva, S., Poscablo, C., Habousha, R. et al. (2012) Mind-body medicine therapies for a range of depression severity: a systematic review. *Psychosomatics*, 53: 407–423.

Figueroa, R. (2010) Use of antidepressants during pregnancy and risk of attention-deficit/hyperactivity disorder in the offspring. *Journal of Developmental & Behavioral Pediatrics*, 31: 641–648.

Fjorback, L. O., Arendt, M., Ornbol, E. et al. (2011) Mindfulness-based stress reduction and mindfulness-based cognitive therapy: a systematic review of randomized controlled trials. *Acta Psychiatric Scandinavia*, 124: 102–119.

Frawley, J., Adams, J., Sibbritt, D. et al. (2013) Prevalence and determinants of complementary and alternative medicine use during pregnancy: results from a nationally representative sample of Australian pregnant women. *Australian and New Zealand Journal of Obstetrics and Gynaecology*, 53: 347–352.

Frawley, J., Sibbritt, D., Broom, A,. et al. (2016) Women's attitudes towards the use of complementary and alternative medicine products during pregnancy. *Journal of Obstetrics and Gynaecology*, 36: 462–467.

Furnham, A. and Lousley, C. (2013) Mental health literacy and the anxiety disorders. *Health*, 5: 521–531.

Goyal, M., Singh, S., Sibinga, E. M. et al. (2014) Meditation programs for psychological stress and well-being: a systematic review and meta-analysis. *JAMA Internal Medicine*, 174: 357–368.

Grossman, J. and Mackenzie, F. J. (2005) The Randomized Controlled Trial: gold standard, or merely standard? *Perspectives in Biology and Medicine*, 48: 516–534.

Gureje, O., Nortje, G., Makanjuola, V. et al. (2015) The role of global traditional and complementary systems of medicine in treating mental health problems. *Lancet Psychiatry*, 2: 168–177.

Hawk, C., Adams, J. and Hartvigsen, J. (2015) The role of CAM in public health, disease prevention, and health promotion. *Evidence-Based Complementary and Alternative Medicine*, 2015: 528487.

Hofmann, S. G., Sawyer, A. T., Witt, A. A. et al. (2010) The effect of mindfulness-based therapy on anxiety and depression: a meta-analytic review. *Journal of Consulting and Clinical Psychology*, 78: 169–183.

Hung, S. K., Perry, R. and Ernst, E. (2011) The effectiveness and efficacy of Rhodiola rosea L.: a systematic review of randomized clinical trials. *Phytomedicine*, 18: 235–244.

Iyengar, B. K. S. (1965) *Light on Yoga*, London: Allen & Unwin.

Jayakody, K., Gunadasa, S. and Hosker, C. (2014) Exercise for anxiety disorders: systematic review. *British Journal of Sports Medicine*, 48(3): 187–196.

Jorm, A. F., Morgan, A. J. and Hetrick, S. E. (2008) Relaxation for depression. *Cochrane Database of Systematic Reviews*, Cd007142.

Leach, M. J. (2016) Does 'traditional' evidence have a place in contemporary complementary and alternative medicine practice? A case against the value of such evidence. *Focus on Alternative and Complementary Therapies*, 21: 147–149.

Lopresti, A.L. and Drummond, P.D. (2014) Saffron (Crocus sativus) for depression: a systematic review of clinical studies and examination of underlying antidepressant mechanisms of action. *Human Psychopharmacology: Clinical and Experimental*, 29: 517–527.

Maher, A.R., Hempel, S., Apaydin, E. et al. (2016) St. John's wort for major depressive disorder: a systematic review. *Rand Health Quarterly*, 5: 12.

Malhi, G. S., Bassett, D., Boyce, P. et al. (2015) Royal Australian and New Zealand College of Psychiatrists clinical practice guidelines for mood disorders. *Australian & New Zealand Journal of Psychiatry*, 49: 1087–1206.

McGuire, T. M., Walters, J. A., Dean, A.J. et al. (2009) *Review of the Quality of Complementary Medicines Information Resources: Summary Report*. Sydney: National Prescribing Service Limited, pp. 1–54.

McHugh, R. K., Whitton, S. W., Peckham, A.D. et al. (2013) Patient preference for psychological vs. pharmacological treatment of psychiatric disorders: a meta-analytic review. *The Journal of Clinical Psychiatry*, 74: 595–602.

McIntyre, E., Saliba, A. J., Wiener, K. K K. et al. (2015) Prevalence and predictors of herbal medicine use in adults experiencing anxiety: A critical review of the literature. *Advances in Integrative Medicine*, 2: 38–48.

McIntyre, E., Saliba, A. J, Wiener, K. K. K. et al. (2016) Herbal medicine use behaviour in Australian adults who experience anxiety: a descriptive study. *BMC Complement Alternative Medicine*, 16: 60.

McIntyre, E., Saliba, A. J., Wiener, K. K K, et al. (2017) Predicting the intention to use herbal medicines for anxiety symptoms: a model of health behaviour. *Journal of Mental Health*, 26: 1–8.McIntyre, R. S., Filteau, M-J., Martin, L. et al. (2014) Treatment-resistant depression: Definitions, review of the evidence, and algorithmic approach. *Journal of Affective Disorders*, 156: 1–7.

Morgan, A. J. and Francis, A. J. P. (2008) Australian natural therapists and mental health: Survey of treatment approaches and referral patterns. *Journal of Complementary and Integrative Medicine*, 5.

Murthy, V., Adams, J., Broom, A, et al. (2017) The influence of communication and information sources upon decision-making around complementary and alternative medicine use for back pain among Australian women aged 60–65 years. *Health & Social Care in the Community*, 25: 114–122.

Nakhai-Pour, H. R., Broy, P. and Bérard, A. (2010) Use of antidepressants during pregnancy and the risk of spontaneous abortion. *CIMAJ : Canadian Medical Association Journal*, 182: 1031–1037.

National Institute for Health and Care Excellence. (2009) *Depression in Adults: Recognition and Management*, London: NICE.

Ng, Q. X., Koh, S.S.H., Chan, H. W. et al. (2017) Clinical use of curcumin in depression: a meta-analysis. *Journal of the American Medical Directors Association*, 18: 503–508.

Opie, R. S, O'Neil, A., Itsiopoulos, C. et al. (2015) The impact of whole-of-diet interventions on depression and anxiety: a systematic review of randomised controlled trials. *Public Health and Nutrition*, 18: 2074–2093.

Pigott, H. E., Leventhal, A. M., Alter, G. S. et al. (2010) Efficacy and effectiveness of antidepressants: current status of research. *Psychotherapy and Psychosomatics*, 79: 267–279.

Pirotta, M., Densley, K., Forsdike, K. et al. (2014) St John's wort use in Australian general practice patients with depressive symptoms: their characteristics and use of other health services. *BMC Complementary and Alternative Medicine*, 14.

Powers, M. B., Zum Vorde Sive Vording, M. B. and Emmelkamp, P. M. (2009) Acceptance and commitment therapy: a meta-analytic review. *Psychotherapy and Psychosomatics*, 78: 73–80.

Reid, R., Steel, A., Wardle, J. et al. (2016) Complementary medicine use by the Australian population: a critical mixed studies systematic review of utilisation, perceptions and factors associated with use. *BMC Complementary Alternative Medicine*, 16: 176.

Rich, J. L., Byrne, J. M., Curryer, C. et al. (2013) Prevalence and correlates of depression among Australian women: a systematic literature review, January 1999–January 2010. *BMC Research Notes*, 6: 424.

Rienks, J., Dobson, A. J. and Mishra, G. D. (2012) Mediterranean dietary pattern and prevalence and incidence of depressive symptoms in mid-aged women: results from a large community-based prospective study. *European Journal of Clinical Nutrition*, 67: 75.

Sarris, J., Gadsden, S. and Schweitzer, I. (2014a) Naturopathic medicine for treating self-reported depression and anxiety: an observational pilot study of naturalistic practice. *Advances in Integrative Medicine*, 1: 87–92.

Sarris, J., Glick, R., Hoenders, R. et al. (2014b) Integrative mental healthcare White Paper: establishing a new paradigm through research, education, and clinical guidelines. *Advances in Integrative Medicine*, 1: 9–16.

Sarris, J., LaPorte, E. and Schweitzer, I. (2011) Kava: a comprehensive review of efficacy, safety, and psychopharmacology. *Australian and New Zealand Journal of Psychiatry*, 45: 27–35.

Sarris, J. and McIntyre, E. (2017) Herbal anxiolytics with sedative actions. In D. Camfield, E. McIntyre and J. Sarris (eds) *Evidence-Based Herbal and Nutritional Treatments for Anxiety in Psychiatric Disorders*, Cham, Switzerland: Springer International Publishing.

Sarris, J., McIntyre, E. and Camfield, D. A. (2013) Plant-based medicines for anxiety disorders, part 2: a review of clinical studies with supporting preclinical evidence. *CNS Drugs*, 27: 301–319.

Sarris, J., Murphy, J., Mischoulon, D. et al. (2016) Adjunctive nutraceuticals for depression: A systematic review and meta-analyses. *American Journal of Psychiatry*, 173: 575–587.

Shreffler-Grant, J., Nichols, E., Weinert, C. et al. (2013) The Montana State University Conceptual Model of Complementary and Alternative Medicine Health Literacy. *Journal of Health Communication*, 18: 1193–1200.

Smith, C A., Hay, P. P. and Macpherson, H. (2010) Acupuncture for depression. *Cochrane Database of Systematic Reviews*, Cd004046.

Solomon, D. and Adams, J. (2015) The use of complementary and alternative medicine in adults with depressive disorders: a critical integrative review. *Journal of Affective Disorders*, 179: 101–113.

Solomon, D., Adams, J. and Graves, N. (2013) Economic evaluation of St. John's wort (Hypericum perforatum) for the treatment of mild to moderate depression. *Journal of Affective Disorders*, 148: 228–234.

Spinks, J. and Hollingsworth, B. (2012) Policy implications of complementary and alternative medicine use in Australia: data from the National Health Survey. *The Journal of Alternative and Complementary Medicine*, 18: 371–378.

Sramek, J. J. and Cutler, N. R. (2011) The impact of gender on antidepressants. In J. C. Neill and J. Kulkarni (eds) *Biological Basis of Sex Differences in Psychopharmacology*, Berlin: Springer, pp. 231–249.

Steel, Z., Marnane, C., Iranpour, C. et al. (2014) The global prevalence of common mental disorders: a systematic review and meta-analysis 1980–2013. *International Journal of Epidemiology*, 43: 476–493.

Taylor, S., Abramowitz, J. S. and McKay, D. (2012) Non-adherence and non-response in the treatment of anxiety disorders. *Journal of Anxiety Disorders*, 26: 583–589.

Walsh, R. and Shapiro, S. L. (2006) The meeting of meditative disciplines and Western psychology: a mutually enriching dialogue. *American Psychology*, 61: 227–239.

Wang, F., Lee, E. K., Wu, T. et al. (2014) The effects of tai chi on depression, anxiety, and psychological well-being: a systematic review and meta-analysis. *International Journal of Behavioral Medicine*, 21: 605–617.

Wardle, J. and Adams, J. (2012) Indirect risks of complementary and alternative medicine. In J. Adams (ed.) *Traditional, Complementary and Integrative Medicine*, Basingstoke: Palgrave, pp. 212–219.

Whiteford, H. A., Buckingham, W. J., Harris, M. G., et al. (2014) Estimating treatment rates for mental disorders in Australia. *Australian Health Review*, 38: 80–85.

Wiles, N., Thomas, L., Abel, A., et al. (2014) Clinical effectiveness and cost-effectiveness of cognitive behavioural therapy as an adjunct to pharmacotherapy for treatment-resistant depression in primary care: the CoBalT randomised controlled trial. *Health Technology Assessment*, 17: 113.

World Health Organization. (2016) Investing in treatment for depression and anxiety leads to fourfold return. Available at: www.who.int/mediacentre/news/releases/2016/depression-anxiety-treatment/en/

World Health Organization. (2017) *Depression and Other Common Mental Disorders; Global Health Estimates*, Geneva: WHO.

# Part III

# CIM use, women and the health care system

# 8 Animating the 'happening' of complementary and integrative medicine

The potential of non-representational theory and some examples through older females' use

*Gavin J. Andrews and Peter N. DeMaio*

## Introduction

Qualitative research examining complementary and integrative medicine (CIM) is well established and scholars of complementary and integrative medicine (CIM) value the rich insights such research can uncover about people's experiences, feelings and opinions. Indeed, while certain studies are focused 'inwardly' on the recognition and progress of qualitative inquiry (Adams et al. 2008), most others are focused 'outwardly' on conveying the empirical world. At one level, consumer issues relating to CIM are a common area of study. Topics such as clients' beliefs, expectations and reasons and decisions with regard to CIM use (Eaves et al. 2015; Lewith and Chan 2002; McLaughlin et al. 2012), their disclosure of use (Robinson and McGrail 2004), their in-treatment decision-making (Bishop et al. 2010) and their overall experiences and outcomes (Alraek and Malterud 2009; Eaves et al. 2015; Luff and Thomas 2000; Magin et al. 2006) have all been studied. At another level, the production side of CIM has been considered by research, including the views, experiences and decisions of therapists, and also how these interact with conventional health services (Adams 2003; 2006; Andrews 2003a; Andrews et al. 2003; McCollum and Gehart 2010).

A general observation that holds true across this broad range of research is that qualitative studies tell us a lot about meaning and identity with respect to CIM. However, arguably what has been largely missed to date is the immediacy of CIM; its happening in space and time materially, performatively and sensorarily (for exceptions, see Barcan 2011; Philo et al. 2015) and this is no less the case for women's health and health care as for other topics regarding CIM.

It is in this literary context and with reference to women's health, and by way of a solution, that this chapter proposes the additional adoption of non-representational theory (NRT) in qualitative research on CIM which can help address these neglects. In terms of structure, the following section introduces NRT. The remainder of the chapter then explores the core interests of NRT one at a time, and the connection of each to CIM. Each of these sections has three aims: (1) to describe the particular area of interest; (2) to discuss elements of CIM and CIM research that align well with it; and (3) to provide a fictional vignette of an older female user's experiences to illustrate NRT in action. The chapter closes with some thoughts on methodological challenges and more broadly on how NRT, contrary to certain critiques, might be suited for researching social intersectionality – such as gender – and the particular situations and challenges experienced by particular groups, such as women.

## The theory of the non-representing, non-representable world

NRT places the raw performance of the world at the centre of inquiries. Broadly speaking, it communicates the many physical, non-verbalized and often automatic, actions and interactions that constitute the majority of everyday life, and how these are acted by humans (and non-humans), picked up by them and affect them (see Thrift 2008). As a way of doing research that speaks to people in their environments, NRT originates from the discipline of human geography. It signifies, however, an obvious departure from the norm for geographers and others who use it. Summarizing past theoretical human geography paradigms: if the early twentieth century was all about the region as a fundamental descriptive unit of analysis (i.e. regional – often 'schoolbook' – geography), the 1950s and 1960s about the spatial patterning of humankind (i.e. positivistic spatial science) and the 1970s to the 1990s onwards all about the structures and meanings of place (i.e. Marxist, humanistic and social constructionist geography), with NRT – arisen partly as a reaction to the pillars of these previous paradigms – the twenty-first century has heralded something quite different again.

Beyond a critique of past paradigms and scholarship, NRT provides its own set of fundamental realizations on what it is to be a human in the world. That humans

> do not always consciously reflect upon external representations – signs, symbols, etc. – when they make sense of the world; that thinking does not necessarily involve the internal manipulation of picture-like representations; that intelligence is a distributed and relational process, in which a range of actors (bodies, texts, devices, objects) are lively participants.
>
> (McCormack 2008: 1824)

Notably 'theory' in NRT is meant as plural (Lorimer 2008). Hence, it does not signify one theory, or a clearly mapped amalgamation of theories. Rather, it describes a number of contact zones between a range of theoretical positions. As Andrews (2014) suggests, NRT brings together ideas from a variety of social science sub-disciplines and fields and draws on varied philosophical approaches and movements (see also Cadman 2009; Vannini 2009). NRT is also selective, drawing out particular arguments from each that serve its purposes the best. Examples include re-reading the works of Derrida and Latour for ideas on the agency, forces and networking of materials, and the works of Merleau-Ponty and

Deleuze for perspectives on pre-consciousness, bodily energy and perceptions and co-evolutions with objects (Cadman 2009).

In sum, the 'non-representational' in NRT can be understood in two ways: one concerning the non-representational world, the other concerned with researching it. On one level, NRT is concerned with how humans live without purposefully representing, i.e. the basic often less-than-fully conscious happenings in life. On another level, NRT is concerned not to re-represent events but instead to 'animate' them and the push of life; a sports media analogy being that, rather than providing post-game analysis, it provides a play-by-play commentary on life's unfolding and performance (McCormack 2013). In terms of perspective, NRT looks for certain things when it engages with the world (see Cadman 2009; Vannini 2009). As suggested, these are outlined in the sections below; their connections to CIM elaborated through a fictional vignette focused upon female users.

## Material, relational assemblages

> Lucy, a retired schoolteacher, is both a cleaner in her local clinic and an occasional client. She is taken by how different it feels at different times of the day in different contexts. When visiting to receive treatment, she is part of an energetic environment where people are coming, going, talking about their treatments and life in general. It's busy, busy, busy, non-stop. When she visits in the evening to clean, however, some key ingredients seem to be missing, which makes the place feel dead. The rooms, facilities and decorations are the same but there are no therapists, no clients, no musical accompaniment, no interactions; just her and her cloths, brooms and liquids, and the sound of clocks quietly ticking . . . tick, tick, tick.
>
> As part of the advice she receives from her therapist, Lucy practises self-care at home and pays close attention to the authenticity of her practice. Important to this authenticity is that she sources herbs from India and China either via post or through friends and family, who have visited these places from time to time. Also important are instructive books and documents, similarly sourced from places where the therapies originated, sometimes many centuries ago. Hence although for Lucy every home session is unique in a sensory sense, through these imports it is strongly informed by and connected to other times and places.

The term assemblage describes what composes events and phenomenon in a way that is not overtly structuralist or essentialist, yet still speaks to their content, order and processual aspects (Marcus and Saka 2006). The idea is that assemblages are 'created' through a process involving the grouping of bodies and objects, and 'actualized' through the release of the potential of these bodies and objects (Duff 2014). Moreover, as Little (2016) argues, the four basic principles of assemblage theory are: (1) social entities are systems composed of ever lesser/smaller elements; (2) elements of a social entity are heterogeneous, with their own character and dynamics and material and expressive roles; (3) any assemblage draws elements from different temporal and spatial scales with their own forces and affects, which help it continually form or deform, and express the same or new forces and affects; and (4) due to its complexity, the behaviour of an assemblage is impossible to

6 G. J. Andrews and P. N. DeMaio

calculate even given extensive knowledge of the elements and their dynamics. NRT does not often, if at all, strictly rehearse the afore-mentioned processes, yet they form a basis for its understandings of, and inquiries into, the happenings in life; scholars ask fundamental questions of assemblages – typically at the outset of studies – such as: What is present? What is arriving? What is leaving? What is passive? What is active? What is interacting, with what and how?

The precedent of assemblage thinking exists in the CIM literature, studies emphasizing different aspects. Doel and Segrott (2004), for example, consider the material components assemblages – signature and supplementary – that help compose and facilitate the taking place of aromatherapy, chiropractic healing and Chinese herbalism. Fox (2013) considers the creativity assemblages in art therapy – 'body-disease-therapist-art-product' – that help produce positive feelings and new capacities in clients. Scott (1998), in the context of homeopathy, thinks about the body as both a biological and expressive entity within an assemblage of other human and non-human actors. Andrews et al. (2013) consider the geographically networked nature of CIM more generally. More theoretically and perhaps more abstractly, scholars have engaged with assemblage theory to fundamentally rethink some core elements of CIM, but at the same time challenge biomedical thinking. Walach (2005), for example, develops quantum explanations for CIM as emerging within complex assemblages that possess non-logical relations, entanglements and movements.

## Virtuality and multiplicity

> Spiritual Life is a large group practice based in a North American city. Because of its size, it is able, through economies of scale, to provide treatments based on the latest technologies, and cater for specialist groups, such as women, older people and children. Therapists, for example, have developed a website dedicated to women's health needs. Content includes 1960s music and images related to women's rights and empowerment useful for home-based music therapy. The website also includes tips on practices in reminiscence therapy for older women, walking them through times and places of their pasts and finding out how they feel about them then and now. Meanwhile sector leadership at Spiritual Life has taken the form of online training for therapists, leading to trademarked practices developed at Spiritual Life rolling out simultaneously across different settings on a regional and even national scale. 'Learn with the therapeutic professionals at Spiritual Life' is the mantra; the tag line repeated on their radio ads playing in kitchens and in cars every morning across the nation.

One facet of NRT is to appreciate virtuality and multiplicity at work in the world. At its most theoretical, this has involved a Deleuzian reading of 'the virtual' as something other than the actual yet still 'real': either surface forces and affects produced by actual events, or a form of potential whereby combinations of forces and affects push forward and are felt, but are not necessarily actualized (Cadman 2009). Moreover, it has involved a Deleuzian reading of 'a multiplicity' as a unique and new complex entity that originates in interactions between simpler/basic elements; an entity that is always in flux and open to inputs/modifications and that can cover space and time. In lay/dictionary terms, however, virtuality (an abstraction or replacement or emulation of a physical event) and multiplicity (a state of being multiple) can equally speak to the way that space-time is ruptured – non-fixed and non-linear – and the relatedness of life across these ruptures (McHugh 2009). As Andrews (2014) describes, whether based on a theoretical or lay reading, virtuality and multiplicity are realized, for example, in things and places that are 'real' to people, yet are not physical or entirely present in space-time and/or multiple happenings that are related, but emerge and co-exist in different spaces-times and/or different happenings in different space-times being experienced in a single space-time.

The precedent of such thinking exists in the CIM literature. In practical terms, there have been a number of studies focused on how the internet – 'cyberspace' – is used to advertise and access therapies (Schmidt and Ernst 2004), and on how visualization is used as a technique to take clients 'elsewhere', for diverse ends such as relaxation, life learning and distraction (Andrews 2004; Andrews and Shaw 2010; 2012). Another example can be found in the literature on music therapy for depression in older adults (e.g., Hanser and Thompson 1994). In this case, the event of listening to music may not have a physical effect in and of itself. However, listening to music from the past is thought to interact with a collection of personal and shared histories from other places and times (both meaningful and affective) which enter and unlock the latent potential of the single space-time therapy event. More generally, Doel and Segrott (2003) consider the diverse materials and practices involved in CIM that create events 'beyond belief'. By this, they mean events that, being more than about cure, relate to consumption and lifestyle urges. Moreover, events that are given an invisible 'push' through their constant marketing via visual and other media.

## Vital bodies and vibrant matter

Emma lost her husband a year ago and has been, quite understandably, grieving for over a year. She has always been gregarious and outgoing, and re-finding this part of her has helped her rebuild her life. She likes clothes; not only quality fabrics which are soft to the touch, but bright colours that she feels radiate her own energy. Emma has returned to wearing these which reflects her return to happiness. She has also joined a walking therapy group. Here she gets to experience nature in a sensory way and feel alive; the wind blowing through the trees, birds flying and singing, water rushing down a hillside. As Emma walks the landscape unfolds, constantly changing. At these times she is not only looking at the landscape but actively reaches for it and is part of it – her booted feet sticking to rocks, her arms reaching for walls and fences, her hands wiping sweat from her brow and her lungs taking in the fresh country air. Emma sometimes stops during a walk to practise her own informal mindfulness techniques, attempting to experience the full physicality of her immediate surroundings in all their glory, clear of cluttering thoughts and her mind's commentary that tends to dwell on her recent loss.

In NRT, vitality is about the aliveness of the living and non-living worlds and their collective potential. With regard to the living, direction is gained specifically from vitalist philosophy, which recognizes the exceptional qualities possessed by organic things; their essential spark and energy, and that they constantly change and evolve (Greenhough 2010). With regard to the non-living, direction is gained from new materialist thinking, particularly the idea of 'vibrant matter', which moves beyond a physics definition of vibration, to describe the capacity of things – from core materials to complexly constructed objects – to act as quasi-agents with their own tendencies, trajectories and forces (Bennett 2009). Both of these lines of thinking recognize that when encounters happen between the living and non-living, an energetic animation results. This is a collective materiality that gives life a range of qualities, including its diversity and spirit, its limitless capacity to develop on its own impulses, and its self-generating continuance and purpose.

In the CIM literature, precedent for such thinking clearly exists and it theoretically underpins broad swathes of practice and research. It has been argued that the attraction and popularity of CIM are related to the power of its underlying shared beliefs; these being in nature, vitalism and spirituality offering clients feelings of empowerment, authenticity and being in-tune with the world (Kaptchuk and Eisenberg 1998). Indeed, these authors claim:

> [V]ital energy takes myriad forms: homeopathy speaks of a 'spiritual vital essence', chiropractic refers to the 'innate' and acupuncture is said to involve the flow of 'qi'. Ayurvedic medicine is based on the power called 'prana', and new age healing practices work with 'psychic' or 'astral' energies. The alternative alliance routinely claims that its methods rely on enhancing 'life forces' as opposed to destroying them with artificial drugs and surgery.
>
> (ibid.: 1062)

One specific example, among many, includes Rubik's (2002) work on 'biofields': complex yet weak electromagnetic fields emanating from organisms – involving the transmission of bioinformation and the regulation of homeodynamics – that account for the holistic effects of much CIM.

## Affective sensations and atmospheres

Meridith regularly attends an art-therapy session at her local community centre, mainly to deal with anxiety she has suffered since entering the menopause. It's not only the expressiveness and meaning of the art that she finds improves her sense of well-being, it's the experience of working together with other people as part of a group. Last Friday she was working on a sculpture and the team got lost in the energy of the experience. Ideas were exchanged with enthusiastic smiling faces, members infectiously leading each other from one task to another, the background music and evening lighting adding to the heady atmosphere. On a recent occasion it was not like this. Meredith was in pain following a minor fall. The team worked enthusiastically as usual but she felt cut off from the energy, unable to give herself up to it. She went home early fearing that she was bringing people down. Thankfully that was a one-off. Meridith is on the mend and looking forward to the next session.

A key facet of NRT is to focus on bodily feelings and sensations, not as personal experiences, but as something 'transpersonal' (Andrews 2014), which has led to the adoption of 'affect' as an explanatory concept (see Anderson 2009; Thrift 2008) – a transitioning of the body and the process whereby it is affected by other bodies, modifies and affects further bodies. This transitioning from one state of the body to another is experiential, it encompasses either an amplification of its energy (i.e. positive affection or a joy/laetitia) or a draining of its energy (i.e. negative affection or a sadness/tristitia) (Deleuze and Parnet 2006). Through providing an energetic uplift (a feeling of potential and possibility) or dampening (a feeling of inertia) affect, this impacts upon well-being primarily in an immediate felt sense, and secondarily through increasing or decreasing involvement in activities that might themselves induce well-being. Importantly, affects are not fully 'known' to or reasoned by people as they occur, but instead are experienced less-than-fully consciously by them.

More broadly, 'affective environments' – the collective expression of affects and their reproduction in places – also register less-than-fully consciously to people, both singularly and collectively, as the prevailing vibe or atmosphere (Anderson 2009). Affective environments might be thought of as distributions of basic feeling but, doing more than this, also as ambient informational modes that allure, modulate attention and invite people to respond. Because of this power, affective environments are often re-produced and spread by public and private interests active at different levels which, through paying attention to the sensory attributes of places often in standardized forms, purposefully seek to provide textures to people's lives which serve their own, often financial, interests (Thrift 2004).

The precedent of such thinking exists in the current CIM literature. Above and beyond a general focus on sensory aspects (see Barcan 2011), a number of studies have considered the role of affect in CIM. Atkinson and Scott (2015), for example, consider the affective energy created in the process of moving and expressing in a school-based and dance movement intervention. Fox (2013) considers how creative practices in art-therapy produce an experimenting flow in bodies and objects which, in turn, produce affects. Philo et al. (2015) consider the affective energy derived from inserting yoga movements and meditation practices into everyday lives, and Andrews et al. (2013) consider the affective energy created by bodies and objects in primary health care-based clinics.

## Impulses and habits

Ella always had difficulty maintaining healthy activities. This was not the case, however, with overeating and smoking brought on by the stress of her late career in PR and advertising; bad habits she undertook automatically in the little breaks she had in her day. Nowadays, however, as she approaches the last few years of her career, and her highest role thus far, she has made some changes for the better. Ella practises yoga and instead of eating and smoking, she fits in a few movements in spaces and moments whenever she can. After a few weeks of doing this, it became her 'go to' action, some-thing that she no longer has to think about or plan. A stretch, a breath in and out, rejuvenating her for the hours ahead.

Impulses and habits are of particular interest in NRT (Dewsbury, 2015; Dewsbury and Bissell, 2015). In terms of basic definitions, while impulses are the biological and/or psychological bodily pushes or urges of varying intensities that might prompt action, habits are the actual repeated actions, ranging from simple move-ments to complex events. In terms of what they do and how they work, either one can be experienced consciously or less-than-fully consciously. Habits might be based on impulses to act in accordance with particular meanings or to experience particular sensations or might be more subtly evoked by the physical or mental feel, familiarity or learning of repetition itself.

Dewsbury and Bissell (2015) argue that understanding impulses challenge scholars to think about: (1) how the very notion of a sovereign, autonomous and willing subject might be flawed, as people and their actions are shaped by wider forces; (2) conversely, how habits might be regarded as a form of intelligence that allows humans to act without conscious effort in familiar situations; (3) how habitual performances and experiences might be one process through which people gain sense, understanding and awareness of the world; and (4) how, in the vitality of life, something new is created and subtracted from habitual performances – something other than and more than what is itself repeated.

The precedent for such thinking exists in mainstream CIM literature. On one level, studies have paid attention to bad/unhealthy habitual practices, such as addictions and compulsive disorders, and what CIM can do to help address these (Atkinson and Scott 2015). On another level, albeit less often, studies have also considered the good/healthy habitual practice of/in CIM itself. Indeed, according to Bishop et al.'s (2010) widely cited operational definition, mindfulness can expand the range of potential experiences subject to individual awareness, and increase emotional awareness of the complexity of cognitive and affective experiences. These aspects of mindfulness are associated with emotional regulation, which is thought to help interrupt cyclical patterns of negative emotions and thoughts (D'Avanzato et al. 2013).

## Foregrounds and backgrounds

Holistic Lives is small group practice in a rural town. The experience of the clinic begins in the waiting room and is continued in each practice space, calming Celtic music or sometimes waves washing, the smell of spiced candles, soft lighting, nature artwork, soft furniture and linen. This is the context to all that goes on in Holistic Lives. In the waiting room, however, when one has not much to do, one's attention might be drawn to a new arrival, a client asking to change an appointment, a phone call and eventually to one's own call. It's a spectacle that passes time, but the general atmosphere remains calm and spiritual where even abrupt events seem less grating, less franticly conducted. The therapists at Holistic Life undertook some basic research and asked their clients what they thought about their facility and services. The findings included many comments from older people, women and children in particular that mentioned the ambient yet vibrant atmosphere which they appreciated and contrasted with the atmospheres of conventional primary health care settings.

NRT is concerned with the overall physical and sensory picture; both the foregrounds and the backgrounds in life. Foregrounds are the happenings and unfoldings that dominate and make a moment, the physicality and conscious registering of: 'accidents, predicaments, advents, transactions, adventures, appearances, turns, calamities, proceedings, celebrations, mishaps, phenomena, ceremonies, coincidences, crises, emergencies, episodes, junctures, milestones, becomings, miracles, occasions, chances, triumphs, and many more' (Vannini 2015b). What are important to foregrounds are the practices and performances that make them up; the expressive arrangement and engagement of bodies and objects, including intervals and spacings between them. These visual geometries might be less-than-fully consciously registered by people, yet still make the world familiar and comprehensible (Thrift 2008).

Backgrounds, meanwhile, are the many things and events that fall outside full awareness, being less-than-fully consciously registered and/or taken for granted in environments, such as lighting, shadows, colours, temperatures, or body and object events, either too far off to discern or not in immediate focus (Vannini 2015b). Backgrounds frame events, yet the term background belies the fact that they possess subtle power helping create affective moods, atmospheres and the energies of places, particularly as they are almost always open to, or result from, some form of manipulation.

The precedent of such thinking exists in the CIM literature in studies of therapeutic design; how attention to indoor and outdoor designs might induce healing experiences (Schweitzer et al. 2004). Elsewhere, other studies, although not specifically design-orientated, have noted how body positioning, textures, lighting, colours and sounds of CIM settings are all critical to therapeutic encounters and overall experiences (Andrews et al. 2013; Doel and Segrott 2004).

## Qualities of movement-space

Marg likes to break her days volunteering in her busy seaside town to visit Fay who practises therapeutic massage and reflexology in a clinic near the seafront. This week Marg comes in for her weekly therapy session in the middle of a particularly busy Wednesday, the streets full of shoppers going about their business, cars passing quickly in constant flows; beeping, accelerating, braking. She walks purposefully and briskly down the street, aiming to get out of the rain. Soon after greeting Marg at the door, Fay leads her into a quiet therapy room and gets to work moving carefully but purposefully in her actions, building a regular rhythm as she goes from one body part to another. The regularity of the motion almost puts Marg to sleep; and the fact that Fay is moving in time with the background music certainly plays its part. After her session is finished, Marg leaves Fay's clinic and steps out onto the road. The session has put her in another head space. The town outside now contrasts. It seems even busier, noisier, more frantic and crazier than before, and now Marg feels decidedly out of place in all of this and a little overwhelmed. She decides to amble home slowly and carry on relaxing.

Thrift (2008) suggests that all life is based on and in movement. In fact, so important is movement to NRT that scholars have attempted to integrate it into fundamental metaphysical thinking about collective life and the progression of the world. Most notably, Merriman (2012) proposes the concept of 'movement-space' as a way of thinking about the on-flow of existence. Movement space incorporates the more familiar idea of 'space-time' (space and time unfolding together) but also a range of other physical and felt qualities which, by dealing directly with the realms of forwardly expelled force, energy and sensation, speak even better to the nature of human practice and experience (as Andrews (2018) suggests, these might include affect, velocity, acceleration, rhythm, momentum, imminence and encounter).

In the CIM literature, rhythm is often thought of in terms of natural bodily processes, for example, the potential of yoga to intervene in biological rhythms such as cortisol levels and mood states at particular stages of disease (Raghavendra et al. 2009). Some precedent of NRT-related thinking exists, however. Studies of yoga have also emphasized the importance of rhythm in its constituent movements (Kenny 2002). Atkinson and Scott (2015) explore how dance movement therapy creates 'smooth spaces' which are open and free, and occupied by intensities and events, that enable therapeutic, well-being experiences (as opposed to life as typically lived across 'striated space' where movement is restricted by categories, rules and codes).

## Conclusion

Engaging with geography is not a new or unusual development in CIM research, including or without a focus upon female users and participants. Geographical ideas and concepts have been applied in CIM studies over many years; this scholarship considers, for example, the distributive features of CIM across space (Adams et al. 2011; Wardle et al. 2011), CIM-related features and trends in particular jurisdictions or regions (Wiles and Rosenberg 2001), and the meaning of place and felt 'sense of place' in practice environments (Andrews 2003b). Following some early empirical reconnaissance and precedent (e.g. Andrews et al. 2013; Atkinson and Scott 2015; Doel and Segrott 2003; 2004; Fox 2013; Philo et al. 2015), the current chapter, however, showcases an application through a new theoretical perspective and research lens. As the chapter illustrates, there is considerable theoretical and empirical alignment between CIM and NRT. Indeed, CIM's immediate physical and sensory happening – its 'taking place' – is an important and absolutely inescapable part of its production and consumption. Hence, employing NRT in CIM research might open up studies to the unconscious, raw performance of CIM and the affective influence this has on its female users.

Adopting NRT in CIM research does not have to follow strict rules or criteria. As Lorimer (2008) suggests, NRT can reverberate in the background of research, producing a style of scholarship that looks at common and important immediacies of life. However, deploying NRT in CIM research certainly requires some degree of methodological adjustment involving revised relationships between researchers, subjects and settings (see Vannini 2015a). Some of these adjustments are based on an overall objective to 'witness' the unfolding of events – to show their showing – so that research findings are faithful to them (see Dirksmeier and Helbrecht 2008). Consistent with its belief in the power of the active world is NRT's methodological dedication to act into life to 'boost' it in positive directions, and to assist the world in speaking up. Practically, this has involved the development of ethnographic 'observant participation', which is about getting involved and invested in the physical effort and experience of a situation, and actively intervening to change the course of events (Dewsbury 2009). Moreover, this has involved the use of arts-based approaches that insert new movements, affects and messages into the world, communicating in different and often more direct and powerful ways to larger and more diverse audiences. Finally, this has involved a commitment to community-orientated public scholarship, particularly where researchers align with, and participate in, activist performance and political action (both art-based approaches and a degree of sectorial advocacy already, of course, being commonplace in CIM research).

Above all, embracing NRT in CIM research involving women's health requires each researcher to develop a particular mindset and disposition; what might be thought of as a form of wonderment or enchantment with the physical world. On a conceptual level, this involves an holistic understanding of existence; that humans are not set apart from the world, but instead are the world, part of its endless cycles of energy and movement, but one manifestation of and in it. On a practical level, this involves resisting the academic urge to immediately dig for meaning when looking at empirical subjects and occurrences, and instead observe life's basic emergence and flows (not unlike an academic form of mindfulness). Such wonderment or enchantment leads to the kinds of afore-mentioned experimental methodologies which realize the parts played by researchers and subjects in greater happenings and their opportunity to experiment with them.

# References

Adams, J. (2003) 'The positive gains of integration: a qualitative study of GPs' perceptions of their complementary practice', *Primary Health Care Research and Development*, 4(2): 155–162.

Adams, J. (2006) 'An exploratory study of complementary and alternative medicine in hospital midwifery: models of care and professional struggle', *Complementary Therapies in Clinical Practice*, 12(1): 40–47.

Adams, J., Broom, A. and Jennaway, M. (2008) 'Qualitative methods in chiropractic research: one framework for future inquiry', *Journal of Manipulative and Physiological Therapeutics*, 31(6): 455–460.

Adams, J., Sibbritt, D., Broom, A. et al. (2011) 'A comparison of complementary and alternative medicine users and use across geographical areas: a national survey of 1,427 women', *BMC Complementary and Alternative Medicine*, 11(1): 85.

Alraek, T. and Malterud, K. (2009) 'Acupuncture for menopausal hot flashes: a qualitative study about patient experiences', *The Journal of Alternative and Complementary Medicine*, 15(2): 153–158.

Anderson, B. (2009). 'Non-representational theory', in *The Dictionary of Human Geography*, Oxford: Oxford University Press, pp. 503–504.

Andrews, G. J. (2003a) 'Nurses who left the British NHS for private complementary medical practice: why did they leave? Would they return?', *Journal of Advanced Nursing*, 41(4): 403–415.

Andrews, G. J. (2003b) 'Placing the consumption of private complementary medicine: everyday geographies of older peoples' use', *Health and Place*, 9(4): 337–349.

Andrews, G. J. (2004) '(Re)thinking the dynamic between healthcare and place: therapeutic geographies in treatment and care practices', *Area*, 36(3): 307–318.

Andrews, G. J. (2014) 'Co-creating health's lively, moving frontiers: brief observations on the facets and possibilities of non-representational theory', *Health and Place*, 30: 165–170.

Andrews, G. J. (2018) *Non-Representational Theory and Health: The Health in Life in Space-Time Revealing*, London: Routledge.

Andrews, G. J., Evans, J. and McAlister, S. (2013) 'Creating the right therapy vibe: relational performances in holistic medicine', *Social Science and Medicine*, 83, 99–109.

Andrews, G. J., Peter, E. and Hammond, R. (2003) 'Receiving money for medicine: some tensions and resolutions for community-based private complementary therapists', *Health and Social Care in the Community*, 11(2): 155–167.

Andrews, G. J., and Shaw, D. (2010) '"So we started talking about a beach in Barbados": visualization practices and needle phobia', *Social Science and Medicine*, 71, 1804–1810.

Andrews, G. J. and Shaw, D. (2012) 'Place visualization: conventional or unconventional practice?', *Complementary Therapies in Clinical Practice*, 18(1): 43–48.

Atkinson, S. J. and Scott, K. E. (2015) 'Stable and destabilised states of subjective wellbeing: dance and movement as catalysts of transition', *Social and Cultural Geography*, 16: 75–94

Barcan, R. (2011) *Complementary and Alternative Medicine: Bodies, Therapies, Senses*, Oxford: Berg.

Bennett, J. (2009) *Vibrant Matter: A Political Ecology of Things*, Durham, NC: Duke University Press.

Bishop, F. L., Yardley, L. and Lewith, G. T. (2010) 'Why consumers maintain complementary and alternative medicine use: a qualitative study', *The Journal of Alternative and Complementary Medicine*, 16(2): 175–182.

Cadman L. (2009) 'Nonrepresentational theory/nonrepresentational geographies', in R. Kitchin and N. Thrift (eds) *International Encyclopedia of Human Geography*, Oxford: Elsevier.

D'Avanzato, C., Joormann, J., Siemer, M. and Gotlib, I. H. (2013) 'Emotion regulation in depression and anxiety: examining diagnostic specificity and stability of strategy use', *Cognitive Therapy and Research*, 37(5): 968–980.

Deleuze, G. and Guattari, F. (1988) *A Thousand Plateaus: Capitalism and Schizophrenia*, London: Bloomsbury Publishing.

Deleuze, G. and Parnet C. (2006) *Dialogues II*, London: Continuum.

Dewsbury, J. D. (2009) 'Performative, non-representational and affect-based research: seven injunctions', in D. Delyser, S. Herbert, S. C. Aitken and M. Crang (eds) *The Sage Handbook of Qualitative Geography*, London: Sage.

Dewsbury, J. D. (2015) 'Non-representational landscapes and the performative affective forces of habit: from "Live" to "Blank"', *Cultural Geographies*, 22(1): 29–47.

Dewsbury, J. D. and Bissell, D. (2015) 'Habit geographies: the perilous zones in the life of the individual', *Cultural Geographies*, 22(1): 21–28.

Dirksmeier, P. and Helbrecht, I. (2008) 'Time, non-representational theory and the "performative turn": towards a new methodology in qualitative social research', *Qualitative Social Research*, 9(2): 1–12.

Doel, M. A. and Segrott, J. (2003). 'Beyond belief? Consumer culture, complementary medicine, and the dis-ease of everyday life', *Environment and Planning D: Society and Space*, 21(6): 739–759.

Doel, M. A. and Segrott, J. (2004) 'Materializing complementary and alternative medicine: aromatherapy, chiropractic, and Chinese herbal medicine in the UK', *Geoforum*, 35(6): 727–738.

Duff, C. (2014) *Assemblages of Health: Deleuze's Empiricism and the Ethology of Life*, Amsterdam: Springer.

Eaves, E. R., Sherman, K. J., Ritenbaugh, C., et al (2015) 'A qualitative study of changes in expectations over time among patients with chronic low back pain seeking four CAM therapies', *BMC Complementary and Alternative Medicine*, 15(1): 12.

Fox, N. J. (2013) 'Creativity and health: an anti-humanist reflection', *Health*, 17(5): 495–511.

Greenhough, B. (2010) 'Vitalist geographies: life and the more-than-human', in B. Anderson and P. Harrison (eds) *Taking Place: Non-Representational Theories and Geography*, Farnham: Ashgate.

Hanser, S. B. and Thompson, L. W. (1994) 'Effects of a music therapy strategy on depressed older adults', *Journal of Gerontology*, 49(6): 265–269.

Kaptchuk, T. J. and Eisenberg, D. M. (1998) 'The persuasive appeal of alternative medicine', *Annals of Internal Medicine*, 129(12): 1061–1065.

Kenny, M. (2002) 'Integrated movement therapy(tm): yoga-based therapy as a viable and effective intervention for autism spectrum and related disorders', *International Journal of Yoga Therapy*, 12(1): 71–79.

Lewith, G. T. and Chan, J. (2002) 'An exploratory qualitative study to investigate how patients evaluate complementary and conventional medicine', *Complementary Therapies in Medicine*, 10(2): 69–77.

Little, D. (2016) Blog. Available at: http://understandingsociety.blogspot.ca/2012/11/assemblage-theory.html

Lorimer, H. (2008) 'Cultural geography: nonrepresentational conditions and concerns', *Progress in Human Geography*, 32(4): 551–559.

Luff, D. and Thomas, K. J. (2000) '"Getting somewhere", feeling cared for: patients' perspectives on complementary therapies in the NHS', *Complementary Therapies in Medicine*, 8(4): 253–259.

Magin, P. J., Adams, J., Heading, G. S., Pond, D. C. and Smith, W. (2006) 'Complementary and alternative medicine therapies in acne, psoriasis, and atopic eczema: results of a qualitative study of patients' experiences and perceptions', *Journal of Alternative and Complementary Medicine*, 12(5): 451–457.

Marcus, G. E. and Saka, E. (2006) 'Assemblage', *Theory, Culture & Society*, 23(2–3): 101–106.

McCollum, E. E. and Gehart, D. R. (2010) 'Using mindfulness meditation to teach beginning therapists therapeutic presence: a qualitative study', *Journal of Marital and Family Therapy*, 36(3): 347–360.

McCormack, D. P. (2008) 'Geographies for moving bodies: thinking, dancing, spaces', *Geography Compass*, 2(6): 1822–1836.

McCormack, D. P. (2013) *Refrains for Moving Bodies: Experience and Experiment in Affective Spaces*, Durham, NC: Duke University Press.

McHugh, K. E. (2009) 'Movement, memory, landscape: an excursion in non-representational thought', *GeoJournal*, 74: 209–218.

McLaughlin, D., Lui, C. W. and Adams, J. (2012) 'Complementary and alternative medicine use among older Australian women: a qualitative analysis', *BMC Complementary and Alter-native Medicine*, 12(1): 34.

Merriman, P. (2012) 'Human geography without time-space', *Transactions of the Institute of British Geographers*, 37(1): 13–27.

Philo, C., Cadman, L. and Lea, J. (2015) 'New energy geographies: a case study of yoga, meditation and healthfulness', *Journal of Medical Humanities*, 36(1): 35–46.

Raghavendra, R. M., Vadiraja, H. S., Nagarathna, R. et al. (2009) 'Effects of a yoga program on cortisol rhythm and mood states in early breast cancer patients undergoing adjuvant radiotherapy: a randomized controlled trial', *Integrative Cancer Therapies*, 8(1): 37–46.

Robinson, A. and McGrail, M. R. (2004) 'Disclosure of CAM use to medical practitioners: a review of qualitative and quantitative studies', *Complementary Therapies in Medicine*, 12(2): 90–98.

Rubik, B. (2002) 'The biofield hypothesis: its biophysical basis and role in medicine', *The Journal of Alternative and Complementary Medicine*, 8(6): 703–717.

Schmidt, K. and Ernst, E. (2004) 'Assessing websites on complementary and alternative medicine for cancer', *Annals of Oncology*, 15(5): 733–742.

Schweitzer, M., Gilpin, L. and Frampton, S. (2004) 'Healing spaces: elements of environmental design that make an impact on health', *Journal of Alternative and Complementary Medicine*, 10(Suppl. 1): S-71.

Scott, A. L. (1998) 'The symbolizing body and the metaphysics of alternative medicine', *Body and Society*, 4(3): 21–37.

Thrift, N. (2004) 'Intensities of feeling: towards a spatial politics of affect', *Geografiska Annaler: Series B, Human Geography*, 86(1): 57–78.

Thrift, N. (2008) *Non-Representational Theory: Space, Politics, Affect*, London: Routledge.

Vannini, P. (2009) 'Nonrepresentational theory and symbolic interactionism: shared perspectives and missed articulations', *Symbolic Interaction*, 32(3): 282–286.

Vannini, P. (2015a) *Non-representational Methodologies: Re-envisioning Research*, London: Routledge.

Vannini, P. (2015b) 'Non-representational research methodologies: an introduction', in P. Vaninni (ed.) *Non-representational Methodologies: Re-envisioning Research*, London: Routledge.

Walach, H. (2005) 'Generalized entanglement: a new theoretical model for understanding the effects of complementary and alternative medicine', *Journal of Alternative and Complementary Medicine*, 11(3): 549–559.

Wardle, J., Adams, J., Magalhães, R. J. S. and Sibbritt, D. (2011) 'Distribution of complementary and alternative medicine (CAM) providers in rural New South Wales, Australia: a step towards explaining high CAM use in rural health?', *Australian Journal of Rural Health*, 19(4): 197–204.

Wiles, J. and Rosenberg, M. W. (2001) '"Gentle caring experience": seeking alternative health care in Canada', *Health and Place*, 7(3): 209–224.

Williams, A. (1998) 'Therapeutic landscapes in holistic medicine', *Social Science and Medicine*, 46(9): 1193–1203.

# 9 Maternity care providers and complementary and integrative medicine

*Amie Steel, Abigail Aiyepola, Jane Frawley and Helen Hall*

## Introduction

Maternity care includes pregnancy, labour and postnatal care and support for women and babies up to six weeks after birth. Depending on their physical and social circumstances, and the options available to them, childbearing women will seek out a variety of health care providers to assist them during this important time, and maternity care operates in a pluralistic environment where women access care and make decisions based on the perceived risks and benefits to themselves and their baby. These decisions may include the use (or not) of complementary and integrative medicine (CIM) for general health during pregnancy as well as pregnancy-related health complaints (Frawley et al. 2014).

This chapter aims to explore the interface between maternity care providers and CIM. First, we overview a paradigm proposed by Davis-Floyd (2001) to understand the approaches different maternity care providers advocate for childbearing women. Then we outline the different health professionals commonly involved in maternity care provision and explore how the Davis-Floyd paradigms may influence the maternity care provider's relationship to CIM. Lastly, we will summarise the attitudes and perceptions towards CIM among maternity care providers based on existing research.

## The three paradigms of childbirth

In 2001, Davis-Floyd proposed three discrete models of healthcare seen as significantly impacting contemporary maternity care: the *technocratic, humanistic* and *holistic models* (Davis-Floyd 2001). Through exploration of these three paradigms, the reader may gain new insights that can relate to and help possibly understand the decision-making of not only maternity care providers but also childbearing women, and perhaps explore how these approaches may align or compare across the woman-provider relationship.

- The *technocratic model*: underpinned by an objective, reductionist approach, this embraces a principle of separation through which childbearing is divided into individual component parts. Through this principle, the birth process is seen as unpredictable and the mother's body viewed as a 'machine' upon which health practitioners use tools and technologies to manipulate childbirth. This view is further reinforced by a perception of the mother requiring outside intervention to address any deficiencies in the childbirth process, rather than embodying a capacity to remedy any issues from within.

- The *humanistic model* emphasises balance and connection and attempts to humanise the childbearing experience through a partnership-oriented perspective which is compassionate and responsive to individual needs. This model acknowledges the mind-body connection and values both subjective and objective findings of clinical examinations. Humanistic pregnancy care providers take into account the woman's biology, psychology and social circumstances.
- The *holistic model* emphasises connection and integration as pre-eminent concepts. This view moves beyond the concept of the woman's body as an organism to embrace the notion of the woman as an energy system. Those practising within this paradigm encourage, indeed require, women to be active and engaged in their birth experience. Providers following the humanistic childbirth model consider themselves equal partners with the pregnant/labouring woman, and that all aspects of the woman (emotional, spiritual, physical, mental, and environmental) are important and must be considered when providing care to childbearing women. It is this latter model which appears to align most closely with the philosophy underpinning much CIM.

Davis-Floyd's models offer a way to perceive pluralistic maternity care beyond simply describing and examining women's access to a range of services and providers. The models offer a useful insight to maternity care, by taking into consideration an ideal-type of different philosophical approaches to childbearing that can be held by women and maternity health professionals. While the Davis-Floyd model does not link specific paradigms to any one health profession, in this chapter we will explore the evidence underpinning any such relationships. Competing viewpoints on childbirth, such as is highlighted by the different paradigms outlined by Davis-Floyd, can have a significant influence upon maternity care provision and women's decision-making in a range of ways and may well influence and help interpret women's use of CIM and consultations with CM practitioners during pregnancy, labour and birth.

## Conventional maternity care providers through the lens of Davis-Floyd

Women with a confirmed pregnancy commonly access the services of a qualified maternity care provider (MCP) (Clark et al. 2015). However, in many cases a number of health care providers, holding potentially varying views, contribute to women's care (Steel et al. 2012; Steel et al. 2016). With this in mind, researching conventional maternity care requires an understanding of the perspectives of the health professionals commonly associated with such maternity care provision. It is important to note that there are regional and jurisdictional variabilities in the structure of maternity services internationally, and these differences manifest in variations in the professions operating within the maternity health workforce (Hanafin and O'Reilly 2012). In some countries, nurses, community health workers (CHWs) and traditional birth attendants (TBAs) are involved in maternity care, while in other geographies women will access the care of an obstetrician and/or a midwife (ibid.). In this chapter, our focus is upon obstetricians and midwives, and examining the potential role of these conventional health care providers in women's use of CIM during pregnancy, labour and birth.

### Obstetricians

Obstetricians are medical doctors who have undertaken specialist training in pregnancy and birth. The definition of obstetric care relates to the health care of women, particularly as it relates to childbirth (Royal Australian and New Zealand College of Obstetricians and Gynaecologists 2011).

While obstetricians do sometimes manage normal pregnancy and birth, they are nevertheless deemed experts in pathologic pregnancy and childbirth (Amelink-Verburg and Buitendijk 2010). We propose the obstetric perspective can be interpreted as generally being based upon a *technocratic* model which is risk-adverse (Healy et al. 2016) and reductionist (Wendland 2007) in nature. As a possible outcome of this model, there is growing evidence that women who consult with an obstretrician as their primary maternity care provider have a much greater rate of obstetric intervention, despite questions as to the necessity of all such interventions (Chandraharan 2014; Dahlen et al. 2013; MacFarlane et al. 2016; Tracy et al. 2014). This interventionist approach can be necessary due to complications (Ensing et al. 2015). In such circumstances, obstetric care reduces the risk of death or illness, for women and babies requiring medical intervention (ibid.). In contrast, concerns have been raised by the World Health Organisation regarding the obstetric management of healthy pregnancies – where no complications exist – which increases the medicalisation of normal birth and may have significant maternal and child health and social consequences (Betran et al. 2016).

The values and perspectives held by an obstetrician aligned with the technocratic paradigm may conflict with women's use of CIM for pregnancy and childbirth. While there is growing evidence of some CIM as both safe and effective (Ding et al. 2013; Steel et al. 2015) in supporting pregnant and birthing women, the philosophies underpinning most CIM emphasise empowerment of the individual, self-care and the support for natural processes (Foley and Steel 2017); all concepts which run counter to the core characteristics of the technocratic model.

### Midwives

In many countries, midwives are the primary health care professionals providing care for healthy childbearing women (Hanafin and O'Reilly 2012). Midwifery philosophy aligns with a *humanistic* model where childbirth is viewed as a physical, social, cultural and emotional experience (Bradfield et al. 2017; Došler and Mivšek 2015). Midwives promote childbearing as a normal life event in most situations (Healy et al. 2016) as they hold a foundational belief in the natural processes and empowerment of women (Bradfield et al. 2017) and the importance of respecting women's choices and preferences (Nieuwenhuijze and Low 2013) through this experience. As such, midwives commonly promote normal birth and are cautious of the over-use of technology (Došler and Mivšek 2015; Sinclair and Gardner 2001). Within the humanistic model, CIM may be considered as providing useful additional tools and techniques within a biomedical framework (Shuval and Gross, 2008), particularly where CIM is preferred by women based on their social and cultural values (Bishop et al. 2007).

There is also a sub-group of the midwifery community which may align even more so with the *holistic* model of pregnancy care. This group, commonly linked with community-based midwifery care, or 'homebirth', is often defined based on their emphasis not only on normality and collaboration with the woman (Kennedy and Shannon 2004), but also their opposition to the perceived 'medicalisation' of birth (Johanson et al. 2002). This perspective is not to be confused with lack of competency in biomedical knowledge and technological skills of modern childbirth, but rather a preference for individualised woman-centred care manifest through deep connection with the woman and intuitive knowledge to inform their clinical decision-making (Davis-Floyd and Davis 1996). As previously described, midwifery practice within a holistic model embraces the view of the woman as an 'energy system'. The application of CIM within the holistic model moves beyond midwives supporting woman-centred care to reflect a shared philosophy with CIM and supporting birth as a natural and energetic process. This view enables midwives to not only integrate CIM with research evidence but also a number of energetic medicines with the broad remit of CIM such as homeopathy (Lenger 2004), flower essences (Cram 2001), and reiki (Macpherson 2014).

## Conventional maternity care providers and women's use of CIM in pregnancy, labour and birth

A body of evidence relating to conventional MCPs' engagement with CIM has grown over the last decade. A review of the literature conducted by Adams et al. (2011) appraised 14 articles via three key themes: (1) prevalence of referral, recommendation and practice of CIM; (2) attitudes and views on CIM; and (3) professionalism and professional identity relating to CIM. In the following section, an overview of the current literature regarding conventional MCPs' use of CIM builds upon this previous review, with an additional eight studies that have been published more recently (Table 9.1).

The findings of the review by Adams et al (2011) suggest that in some situations MCPs may practise, endorse or refer women to CIM in the maternity setting. The authors identified a wide range of CIM modalities used by MCPs (ibid.). However, there may be significant variations of CIM use by MCPs in geographical locations,

Table 9.1 Research articles examining health professionals' perceptions of CIM use by women during pregnancy, labour and birth (PLB)

| Author/Year | Sample (size) | Country | Method | CIM investigated |
|---|---|---|---|---|
| Hall, Griffiths and McKenna (2013) | Midwives (n = 25) | Australia | Interviews and observations | Any CIM |
| Hunter (2012) | Doulas (n = 9) | United States | Ethnography (observation and interviews) | Doula care |
| Koc, Topatan and Saglam (2012) | Midwives (n = 129) | Turkey | Survey | Any CIM |
| Mullin et al. (2011) | Midwives (n = 187) | United States | Survey | Chiropractic |
| Samuels et al. (2013) | Obstetricians (n = 170) | Israel | Survey | Any CIM |
| Smith et al. (2005) | Naturopaths (n = 110) | Australia | Survey | Naturopathy |
| Stevens et al. (2011) | Midwives (n = 12); Doulas (n = 6) | Australia | Focus groups | Doula care |
| Williams and Mitchell (2007) | Heads of Maternity Services (n = 60) | England | Semi-structured questionnaire | Aromatherapy |

which may be affected by the presence of CIM within the broader health system as well as larger social and cultural contexts (Bishop and Lewith 2010; Bishop et al. 2007). The 2011 review also suggests more alignment between CIM and midwifery rather than obstetrics, with women in midwife-led models of care more likely to have CIM recommended to them, compared to those in obstetric models of care (Adams et al. 2011). According to the 2011 review, the specific CIM supported by obstetricians and midwives also differed; obstetricians were more likely to refer women to use acupuncture or vitamin supplements, while midwives tend to endorse massage, yoga and aromatherapy. However, it was acknowledged that as women often instigate their own engagement with CIM prior to discussions with MCPs, CIM commonly used by childbearing women and CIM recommended by MCPs may differ.

## Approach of conventional maternity health professionals to CIM use in pregnancy and childbirth

Adams et al. (2011) reported MCPs, particularly midwives, place high value upon CIM as a supplement to antenatal and intra-partum care. A qualitative study of midwifery managers (Williams and Mitchell 2007) appears to support this conclusion, with participants reporting CIM benefits for women such as providing options when conventional medicine proves insufficient. Although the midwifery managers did identify that CIM improved pregnant women's physical and mental health, this was not the central focus to the rationale provided for the use of CIM by pregnant and birthing woman and was also the only reference to health factors given by the study participants (ibid.). This may suggest that the worth placed on CIM by midwives relates to a perceived role of supporting the values of midwifery, as much as it relates to the woman's health. As possible evidence of this, the midwifery managers from this 2007 study also expressed benefits for midwives when CIM is integrated into care for pregnant women, including job satisfaction, extended repertoire of available health care options and the personal sense of reward gained from promoting normality and woman-centred care. Beyond benefits for both midwives and women, Williams and Mitchell also explored the constraints of CIM integration into the conventional maternity care setting perceived by midwifery managers. These which were broadly categorised as: lack of resources, both fiscal and human; influence of organisation and colleagues; and lack of an evidence base. As a barrier, the influence of organisations and colleagues related to a need to provide equitable service to all women and consequently only make CIM treatments available within the maternity unit if they could be offered through 24-hour service. This barrier was argued by the study participants to be further compounded by bureaucratic requirements necessary to allow private CIM practitioners to service women within the maternity unit as well as a concurrent lack of CIM knowledge among midwives in the practice setting. Finally, the lack of an evidence base was described by study participants as a multi-faceted constraint. The lack of scientific research investigating the safety and efficacy of CIM in pregnancy and childbirth is an obvious facet to this perceived barrier, however, the participants in the Williams and Mitchell (2007) study also identified a lack of regulation of CIM, and inconsistent training of CIM practitioners as other aspects affecting the evidence base of CIM for pregnancy and childbirth. Similar to the constraints described in this study, Adams et al. (2011) have also identified a lack of knowledge and training, and a lack of acceptance by colleagues as factors which minimised practice or referral to CIM practitioners among midwives.

Another qualitative study which extends the review by Jon Adams et al. (2011) explored the attitudes and behaviour of Australian midwives (n = 25) with regards to the use of CIM by pregnant women (Hall et al. 2013b). The findings from this study show that midwives aim to work with women to individualise their maternity care, and minimise the risks associated with childbearing. While many midwives in this study were supportive of CIM, even those who were ambivalent would usually advocate for the women's right to make her own informed decision relating to CIM use, on the proviso that it was safe. According to these midwives, this commitment to supporting informed shared decision-making with women holds equally for women who choose to access CIM as for those that do not. As such, these midwives present their role not as advocates for CIM but as advocates for women's right to choose the most suitable care options during their PLB and to work closely with women to ensure safety. However, the ability of midwives to maintain and fulfil this practice approach to CIM also requires overcoming conflicts in their professional role and authority – particularly when faced with possible opposition from colleagues, such as obstetricians (Hall et al. 2012). Despite their attitudes towards CIM, the study participants in Hall et al.'s study indicated that the practice of midwives in daily routine care was mediated by their professional context. They also showed that as most midwives worked in an environment dominated by biomedicine – a paradigm aligned with the *technocratic* model of healthcare – midwives' support for CIM was often constrained even in those cases where a women's interest in CIM was considered by the midwife to be a safe option.

Beyond these results, Adams et al. (2011) showed midwives more commonly viewed CIM as a safe, natural and useful supplement to conventional treatment when compared to the perspective of obstetricians. This difference in views between the two professions may be influenced by characteristics linked with the different models described by Davis-Floyd (2001). For example, it is possible that obstetricians are more critical of the evidence base of CIM, in line with the technocratic model of childbirth, whereas midwives may place a comparatively higher value on women's preferences or knowledge gathered from experience as well as scientific research (Hall et al. 2013a) in alignment with the humanistic or holistic model. Within the obstetric profession, however, Adams et al. (2011) did suggest that female obstetricians were more likely to hold a positive view of CIM than their male colleagues. However, the degree to which CIM may be exerting influence in this way on the attitudes and behaviours of female obstetricians in a male-dominated workforce (Seltzer 1999) remains unexamined.

## Use of CIM practitioners by women during pregnancy, labour and birth

A study of a large, nationally representative sample of Australian women who had recently given birth was published in 2012 and provided the first examination of consultancy patterns across conventional maternity care providers and CIM practitioners during pregnancy (Steel et al. 2012). The study presented four key findings. First, the study revealed a substantial level of CIM practitioner use, with nearly half of the pregnant women consulting a CIM practitioner concurrent to conventional maternity care providers.

Second, within the wider pattern of concurrent care, the study identified a more complex relationship between the two broader provider groups – consultation with some CIM practitioners (e.g. acupuncturists) was associated with less frequent visits to GPs. It is possible that this finding reflects a change in women's health-seeking behaviour as a result of what they perceive as a discouraging response by their GPs to their concerns or preferences (Adams 2000). It may also highlight a discord between what pregnant women seek (Adams et al. 2009) and what some GPs may consider unhelpful or irrelevant (Joos et al. 2011). Alternatively, this finding may be due to a perception among these pregnant women that GPs are not core to their maternity care needs (instead addressing such needs via CIM practitioners), although some models of care do not require more than one visit with a GP and previous research suggests that the majority of CIM providers are unlikely to discourage women from consulting with a GP (Ben-Arye et al. 2007).

Third, women who reported frequently consulting with a midwife were more likely to consult acupuncturists and doulas, i.e. birth companions. This finding supports previous research identifying midwives as a popular source of CIM information for pregnant women (Adams et al. 2009) and often encouraging CIM use for women in their care (Adams 2006; Hall et al. 2013a). Alternatively, this finding could suggest that women choosing different models of maternity care also hold different values and approaches to CIM use, an issue identified in more general CIM use research (Adams et al. 2003) but still requiring further investigation in relation to maternity care (Honda and Jacobson 2005). There is significant synergy between midwifery and CIM philosophy (Hall et al. 2013a; Hall et al. 2013b) and research identifies midwives as recommending women consult with a range of CIM practitioners (Adams et al. 2011; Hall et al. 2013a). The positive correlation between women's use of CIM and their engagement with midwifery care as reported in the literature to date may be explained by the various political and cultural contexts affecting CIM (e.g. political legitimacy) and midwifery (e.g. structure of maternity care provision) across different health systems, particularly within the context of the Davis-Floyd models of maternity care whereby the *holistic* model of CIM aligns more closely to the *humanistic* approach of midwifery compared to the *technocratic* model of obstetrics.

Fourth, the analysis of consultation patterns for the management of specific pregnancy-related conditions suggests pregnant women are making discretionary decisions regarding whom to consult depending on their immediate health concerns. Chiropractors are frequently consulted for back pain and sciatica, massage therapists consulted more commonly for neck pain, and naturopaths and acupuncturists more likely to be consulted for pregnancy-related nausea (Steel et al. 2012). Women are consulting with CIM practitioners most commonly for management of pain-related conditions. This may be due to women's perceptions of CIM treatments as safer (while being equally effective) than conventional pain management (Adams et al. 2009). In particular, women's concerns regarding the teratogenicity of some pharmaceutics, may be influencing their decision to seek out alternative treatment options. However, this perception is only held when the condition is self-assessed as low risk to them or their babies and women are only rarely consulting with CIM practitioners for more serious complications (Adams et al. 2009). This is consistent with the midwifery approach which defaults to the biomedical, *technocratic* model if the woman's pregnancy becomes complicated (Hall et al. 2013b). Attempts to complement conventional treatments with the care of other therapists still occur – we identified a substantial rate of concurrent CIM and conventional practitioner use among pregnant women with gestational diabetes – and this may be the result of women seeking an improved prognosis for these serious conditions or a more active role in maintaining their health (Adams et al. 2009).

The results of this 2012 study highlight a substantial level of CIM practitioner use during pregnancy and a pattern of selective use across different CIM practitioner groups for different health conditions (Steel et al. 2012). The study findings illustrate the inconsistent relationship between the available clinical evidence and the CIM practitioners used by pregnant women. While there is partial alignment between some of the CIM practitioners consulted and the limitations in the volume of existing clinical evidence, there are also a number of women consulting CIM practitioners for specific conditions despite an absence of clinical evidence. This underlines concerns that women may be accessing unsafe and ineffective practices. In order to help inform safe, effective and coordinated maternity care that reflects the full breadth of practitioner consultations among pregnant women, future research must include examination of decision-making and communication between pregnant women and their maternity care providers about CIM practitioner use. The absence of sufficient clinical evidence regarding many commonly used CIM practices during pregnancy also requires urgent attention.

## Facilitating inter-professional collaboration between health practitioners providing care to pregnant women

Inter-professional communication is core to effective collaboration, however, dynamics which are known to affect the interface between conventional medicine and CIM are suggested to commonly prevent inter-professional communication in health care (O'Daniel and Rosenstein 2008). These barriers include hierarchy (Vickers 2001), historical inter-professional rivalries (Baer 2008), differences in language and jargon (Caspi et al. 2000), variance in levels of qualifications and status (Wardle et al. 2012), and intra-professional differences in practice standards and requirements (Wardle et al. 2013). While some of these barriers are immutable (i.e. historical rivalry between CIM and conventional medicine), issues such as varying levels of qualification and training, and differences in language and jargon may be transformed through effective professional development and education (Steel and Adams 2012). However, to explain the potential overarching influence of differences in models of childbirth for the range of practitioners potentially involved in the care of the same woman, an understanding of Davis-Floyd's model should not be dismissed. As some of the greatest risk of CIM occurs from CIM practitioners failing to refer, or being unable to identify when to refer, to other practitioners (Wardle and Adams 2012), breaking down barriers to inter-professional collaboration and building bridges between CIM and conventional practitioners irrespective of the childbirth model held by each individual practitioner may have a positive effect on patient safety among women who use CIM in maternity care.

Despite the interface between CIM and conventional maternity care providers attracting the attention of researchers (Adams 2006; Adams et al. 2011; Hall et al. 2012; Hall et al. 2013a; Hall et al. 2013b; Steel and Adams 2011 2012; Steel et al. 2012), there is only emerging work which has explored the 'grassroots' communication and collaboration between these two categories of health professionals (Diezel et al. 2013; Steel et al. 2013). This preliminary research has examined the inter-professional communication patterns between CAM practitioners and midwives from the perspective of practising midwives. The study describes low rates of formal communication, although the midwives in the study reported being more likely to initiate formal communication with a CIM practitioner about a woman under the care of both health professionals, rather than receiving formal communication from a CIM practitioner. The reasons for this low rate of CIM practitioner-initiated formal communication may be linked to the 'outsider' status of CIM practice within the maternity care system; a status in part developed through the content of education courses for CIM which emphasise the separation of CIM from the centralised biomedical health services (Vickers 2001). This status may then be reinforced and maintained by the realities of CIM practice which continue to operate outside of state-authorised health care provision (Wardle 2016).

## Conclusion

All health professionals, whether providing conventional maternity care services, practising CIM or integrating the three paradigms described by Davis-Floyd (2001), will benefit from awareness of the trends of healthcare pluralism within maternity care identified in this chapter. Primarily, there is the potential for women to be exposed to diverse, and in some cases conflicting, childbirth models as a result of consulting with a conventional and CIM maternity care provider. In fact, with one in two women consulting with a CIM practitioner during pregnancy, it is likely that another practitioner involved in a woman's maternity care may be a CIM practitioner and as such may be practising outside of the conventional maternity care system.

## References

Adams, J. (2000) 'General practitioners, complementary therapies and evidence-based medicine: the defence of clinical autonomy', *Complementary Therapies in Medicine*, 8(4): 248–52.

Adams, J. (2006) 'An exploratory study of complementary and alternative medicine in hospital midwifery: models of care and professional struggle', *Complementary Therapies in Clinical Practice*, 12(1): 40–7.

Adams, J., Easthope, G. and Sibbritt, D. (2003) 'Exploring the relationship between women's health and the use of complementary and alternative medicine', *Complementary Therapies in Clinical Practice*, 11(3): 156–8.

Adams, J., Lui, C.-W., Sibbritt, D., et al. (2011) 'Attitudes and referral practices of maternity care professionals with regard to complementary and alternative medicine: an integrative review', *Journal of Advanced Nursing*, 67(3): 472–83.

Adams, J., Lui, C.-W., Sibbritt, D., et al. (2009) 'Women's use of complementary and alternative medicine during pregnancy: a critical review of the literature', *Birth*, 36(3): 237–45.

Amelink-Verburg, M. P. and Buitendijk, S. E. (2010) 'Pregnancy and labour in the Dutch maternity care system: what is normal? The role division between midwives and obstetricians', *Journal of Midwifery & Women's Health*, 55(3): 216–25.

Baer, H. (2008) 'The emergence of integrative medicine in Australia: the growing interest of biomedicine and nursing in complementary medicine in a Southern developed society', *Medical Anthropology Quarterly*, 22(1): 52–66.

Ben-Arye, E., Scharf, M. and Frenkel, M. (2007) 'How should complementary practitioners and physicians communicate? A cross-sectional study from Israel', *Journal of the American Board of Family Medicine*, 20(6): 565–71.

Betran, A., Torloni, M., Zhang, J. and Gülmezoglu, A. (2016) 'WHO statement on caesarean section rates', *BJOG: An International Journal of Obstetrics & Gynaecology*, 123(5): 667–70.

Bishop, F. L. and Lewith, G. T. (2010) 'Who uses CAM? A narrative review of demographic characteristics and health factors associated with CAM use', *Evidence-Based Complementary and Alternative Medicine*, 7(1): 11–28.

Bishop, F. L., Yardley, L. and Lewith, G. T. (2007) 'A systematic review of beliefs involved in the use of complementary and alternative medicine', *Journal of Health Psychology*, 12(6): 851–67.

Bradfield, Z., Duggan, R., Hauck, Y. and Kelly, M. (2017) 'Midwives being "with woman": an integrative review', *Women and Birth*. doi:10.1016/j.wombi.2017.07.011.

Caspi, O., Bell, I., Rychener, D., Gaudet, T. and Weil, A. (2000) 'The Tower of Babel: communication and medicine: an essay on medical education and complementary-alternative medicine', *Archives of Internal Medicine*, 160(21): 3193–5.

Chandraharan, E. (2014) 'Fetal scalp blood sampling during labour: is it a useful diagnostic test or a historical test that no longer has a place in modern clinical obstetrics?', *BJOG: An International Journal of Obstetrics & Gynaecology*, 121(9): 1056–62.

Clark, K., Beatty, S. and Reibel, T. (2015) 'Maternity care: a narrative overview of what women expect across their care continuum', *Midwifery*, 31(4): 432–7.

Cram, J. R. (2001) 'Effects of two flower essences on high intensity environmental stimulation and EMF', *Subtle Energies & Energy Medicine Journal Archives*, 12(3): 249–70.

Dahlen, H. G., Schmied, V., Dennis, C.-L. and Thornton, C. (2013) 'Rates of obstetric intervention during birth and selected maternal and perinatal outcomes for low risk women born in Australia compared to those born overseas', *BMC Pregnancy and Childbirth*, 13(1): 100.

Davis-Floyd, R. (2001) 'The technocratic, humanistic, and holistic paradigms of childbirth', *International Journal of Gynecology & Obstetrics*, 75 (Suppl. 1): S5–S23.

Davis-Floyd, R. and Davis, E. (1996) 'Intuition as authoritative knowledge in midwifery and homebirth', *Medical Anthropology Quarterly*, 10(2): 237–69.

Diezel, H., Steel, A., Wardle, J. and Johnstone, K. (2013) 'Patterns and influences of inter-professional communication between midwives and CAM practitioners: a preliminary examination of the perceptions of midwives', *Australian Journal of Herbal Medicine*, 25(1): 4–10.

Ding, M., Leach, M. and Bradley, H. (2013) 'The effectiveness and safety of ginger for pregnancy-induced nausea and vomiting: a systematic review', *Women and Birth*, 26(1): e26–e30.

Došler, A. J. and Mivšek, A. P. (2015) 'Does midwifery philosophy affect perceptions of students regarding female reproduction?', *Health Sociology Review*, 24(2): 175–85.

Ensing, S., Abu-Hanna, A., Schaaf, J. M., Mol, B. W. J. and Ravelli, A. C. (2015) 'Trends in birth asphyxia, obstetric interventions and perinatal mortality among term singletons: a nationwide cohort study', *The Journal of Maternal-Fetal & Neonatal Medicine*, 28(6): 632–7.

Foley, H. and Steel, A. (2017) 'The nexus between patient-centered care and complementary medicine: allies in the era of chronic disease?', *The Journal of Alternative and Complementary Medicine*, 23(3): 158–63.

Frawley, J., Adams, J., Broom, A., et al. (2014) 'Majority of women are influenced by nonprofessional information sources when deciding to consult a complementary and alternative medicine practitioner during pregnancy', *The Journal of Alternative and Complementary Medicine*, 20(7): 571–7.

Hall, H., Griffiths, D. L. and McKenna, L. G. (2012) 'Complementary and alternative medicine in midwifery practice: managing the conflicts', *Complementary Therapies in Clinical Practice*, 18(2012): 246–51.

Hall, H. G., Griffiths, D. L. and McKenna, L. G. (2013a) 'Navigating a safe path together: a theory of midwives' responses to the use of complementary and alternative medicine', *Midwifery*, 29(7): 801–8.

Hall, H., McKenna, L. G. and Griffiths, D. L. (2013b) 'Contextual factors that mediate midwives' behaviour towards pregnant women's use of complementary and alternative medicine', *European Journal of Integrative Medicine*, 5(2013): 68–74.

Hanafin, S. and O'Reilly, E. (2012) 'National and international review of literature on models of care across selected jurisdictions to inform the development of a National Strategy for Maternity Services in Ireland'. Available online at: http://health.gov.ie/wp-content/uploads/2016/01/Literature-review-on-maternity-models-of-care.pdf (accessed 20 July 2016).

Healy, S., Humphreys, E. and Kennedy, C. (2016) 'Midwives' and obstetricians' perceptions of risk and its impact on clinical practice and decision-making in labour: an integrative review', *Women and Birth*, 29(2): 107–16.

Honda, K. and Jacobson, J. (2005) 'Use of complementary and alternative medicine among United States adults: the influences of personality, coping strategies, and social support', *Preventive Medicine*, 40(1): 46–53.

Johanson, R., Newburn, M. and Alison, M. (2002) 'Has the medicalisation of childbirth gone too far?', *British Medical Journal*, 324(7342): 892–5.

Joos, S., Musselmann, B. and Szecsney, J. (2011) 'Integration of complementary and alternative medicine into family practices in Germany: results of a national survey', *Evidence-Based Complementary and Alternative Medicine*, 2011. doi:10.1093/ecam/nep019.

Kennedy, H. P. and Shannon, M. T. (2004) 'Keeping birth normal: research findings on midwifery care during childbirth', *Journal of Obstetric, Gynecologic, & Neonatal Nursing*, 33(5): 554–60.

Koc, Z., Topatan, Z. and Saglam, S. (2012) 'Determination of the usage of complementary and alternative medicine among pregnant women in the Northern Region of Turkey', *Collegian*.

Lenger, K. (2004) 'Homeopathic potencies identified by a new magnetic resonance method: homeopathy: an energetic medicine', *Subtle Energies & Energy Medicine Journal Archives*, 15(3): 225–43.

MacFarlane, A., Blondel, B., Mohangoo, A., et al. (2016) 'Wide differences in mode of delivery within Europe: risk-stratified analyses of aggregated routine data from the Euro-Peristat study', *BJOG: An International Journal of Obstetrics & Gynaecology*, 123(4): 559–68.

Macpherson, J. (2014) *Women and Reiki: Energetic/Holistic Healing in Practice* (1st ed.). New York: Routledge.

Nieuwenhuijze, M. and Low, L. K. (2013) 'Facilitating women's choice in maternity care', *The Journal of Clinical Ethics*, 24(3): 276–82.

O'Daniel, M. and Rosenstein, A. H. (2008) *Professional Communication and Team Collaboration*, Rockville, MD: Agency for Healthcare Research and Quality.

Royal Australian and New Zealand College of Obstetricians and Gynaecologists (2011) 'About the specialty'. Available online at www.ranzcog.edu.au/the-ranzcog/about-specialty.html (accessed 17 July 2013).

Seltzer, V. L. (1999) 'Changes and challenges for women in academic obstetrics and gynecology', *American Journal of Obstetrics and Gynecology*, 180(4): 837–48.

Shuval, J. T., and Gross, S. E. (2008) 'Nurses and midwives in alternative health care: comparative processes of boundary re-configuration in Israel', in J. Adams and P. Tovey (eds), *Complementary and Alternative Medicine in Nursing and Midwifery: Towards a Critical Social Science*, London: Routledge pp. 113–133.

Sinclair, M. and Gardner, J. (2001) 'Midwives' perceptions of the use of technology in assisting childbirth in Northern Ireland', *Journal of Advanced Nursing*, 36(2): 229–36.

Smith, C., Martin, K., Hotham, E. et al. (2005) 'Naturopaths' practice behaviour: provision and access to information on complementary and alternative medicines', *BMC Complementary and Alternative Medicine*, 5: 15.

Steel, A. and Adams, J. (2011) 'The role of naturopathy in pregnancy, labour and postnatal care: broadening the evidence-base', *Complementary Therapies in Clinical Practice*, 17(4): 189–92.

Steel, A. and Adams, J. (2012) 'Developing midwifery and complementary medicine collaboration: the potential of interprofessional education?', *Complementary Therapies in Clinical Practice*, 18(4): 261–4.

Steel, A., Adams, J., Frawley, J. et al. (2016) 'Does Australia's health policy environment create unintended outcomes for birthing women?', *Birth*, 43(4): 273–6.

Steel, A., Adams, J., Sibbritt, D. and Broom, A. (2015) 'The outcomes of complementary and alternative medicine use among pregnant and birthing women: current trends and future directions', *Women's Health*, 11(3): 309–23.

Steel, A., Adams, J., Sibbritt, D., et al. (2012) 'Utilisation of complementary and alternative medicine (CAM) practitioners within maternity care provision: results from a nationally representative cohort study of 1,835 pregnant women', *BMC Pregnancy Childbirth*, 12: 146.

Steel, A., Diezel, H., Wardle, J. and Johnstone, K. (2013) 'Patterns of inter-professional communication between complementary and conventional practitioners providing maternity care services: a preliminary examination of the perceptions of CAM practitioner', *Australian Journal of Herbal Medicine*, 25(2): 57–61.

Stevens, J., Dahlen, H., Peters, K. and Jackson, D. (2011) 'Midwives' and doulas' perspectives of the role of the doula in Australia: a qualitative study', *Midwifery*, 27(4): 509–16.

Tracy, S. K., Welsh, A., Hall, B. et al. (2014) 'Caseload midwifery compared to standard or private obstetric care for first time mothers in a public teaching hospital in Australia: a cross-sectional study of cost and birth outcomes', *BMC Pregnancy and Childbirth*, 14(1): 46.

Vickers, A. J. (2001) 'Message to complementary and alternative medicine: evidence is a better friend than power', *BMC Complementary and Alternative Medicine*, 1: 1.

Wardle, J. (2016) 'Complementary and integrative medicine: the black market of health care?', *Advances in Integrative Medicine*, 3(3): 77–8.

Wardle, J. and Adams, J. (2012) 'Indirect risks of complementary and alternative medicine', in J. Adams, G. J. Andrews, J. Barnes, A. Broom, and P. Magin (eds), *Traditional Complementary and Integrative Medicine: An International Reader*, Basingstoke: Palgrave Macmillan, pp. 212–19.

Wardle, J. L., Adams, J., Lui, C.-W. and Steel, A. E. (2013) 'Current challenges and future directions for naturopathic medicine in Australia: a qualitative examination of perceptions and experiences from grassroots practice', *BMC Complementary and Alternative Medicine*, 13: 15.

Wardle, J., Steel, A. and Adams, J. (2012) 'A review of tensions and risks in naturopathic education and training in Australia: a need for regulation', *The Journal of Alternative and Complementary Medicine*, 18(4): 363–70.

Wendland, C. L. (2007) 'The vanishing mother: Cesarean section and "evidence-based obstetrics"', *Medical Anthropology Quarterly*, 21(2): 218–33.

Williams, J. and Mitchell, M. (2007) 'Midwifery managers' views about the use of complementary therapies in the maternity services', *Complementary Therapies in Clinical Practice*, 13(2): 129–35.

# 10 The role and influence of women in the workforce and practice of complementary and integrative medicine

## Contemporary trends and future prospects

*Jon Adams, David Sibbritt, Jason Prior, Irena Connon, Erica McIntyre, Roger Dunston, Romy Lauche and Amie Steel*

## Introduction

While researchers have examined the consumption of complementary and integrative medicine (CIM) as a social movement inspiring potential social change (e.g. Goldner 2004), the practice of CIM can also be approached and evaluated in the same manner. As this chapter identifies, a small but significant body of literature has explored the synergy and relationship between women's role in CIM practice, gender and the possibility of resisting the dominant biomedical model of health (Nissen 2011).

The broad range of CIM modalities are increasingly acknowledged as constituting a significant component of (primary) health care provision (Grace 2012; Wardle and Adams 2012) and many CIM provider groups, to varying degrees, are seeking elevated status as health care professions (Welsh et al. 2004). Such a process of professionalization (Abbott 1988) involves acquiring jurisdiction or exclusive control over a content of work (Friedson 1970) and gaining legitimacy from the state (Smith-Cunnien 1998) which directly relate to and impact upon the contemporary CIM health workforce.

Meanwhile, the role of women in CIM practitioner ranks is one dynamic important to the current CIM workforce and its future potential. As we identify in this chapter, early work has examined the relationship between CIM and gender (Doel and Segrott 2003; Flesch 2007, 2010; Nissen 2011; Scott 1998), and CIM use and practice raise a number of interesting issues with regards to the role of women in the care of others (provider) and the nature and provision of services provided (professional projects). This chapter examines the role and significance of women across the CIM workforce and practice and explores the contemporary environment relating to CIM in high-income countries that may help facilitate or challenge what some scholars and commentators have interpreted as a 'feminist' CIM approach to health care.

## Women, biomedicine and the conventional medical workforce

It has long been acknowledged that the biomedical model of health and conventional structures of health care delivery explicitly or implicitly help maintain paternalistic power dimensions (Riska and Wegar 1993). Furthermore, commentators have highlighted how clinical trials (Schiebinger 2003), the broader medical and health research enterprise (Inhorn and Whittle 2001) and the recent focus upon evidence-based medicine (Rogers 2004) all contain a number of biases against women (both as providers and receivers of health care).

Indeed, an international body of research has examined aspects of women's involvement in conventional medical practice and health care, revealing a number of interesting findings (Gjerberg 2001; Hojat et al. 2000; Heiligers and Hingstman 2000; Riska 2001). Empirical data suggests that while the gender composition of medicine is changing – with increasing numbers of female medical students identified – the medical profession remains male-dominated (Kilminster et al. 2007). Nevertheless, researchers and commentators have identified what they see as the increasing 'feminization' of medicine and have pondered a number of potential negative and positive consequences of increasing numbers of women moving into medical careers (Levinson and Lurie 2004).

With regards to the Australian context, an Australian Institute of Health and Welfare Workforce Report conducted in 2015 revealed that 40.1 per cent of the medical workforce was female, up from 32.9 per cent in 2005 (AIHW 2016). This report also revealed that the distribution of female practitioners was concentrated in specific areas of practice such as general paediatrics, geriatric medicine and anatomical pathology and the distribution of working hours is on average lower for women than men, with women often more likely to work part-time (34 hours or less per week) and less women working 50 hours or more per week (AIHW 2016). Meanwhile, other Australian data (AIHW 2012, 2013, 2014) reports a majority of physiotherapists (68.8 per cent), psychologists (76.7 per cent) and nurses (90 per cent) as being female – workforce trends generally in line with most other high-income countries (Hammond 2009; Kell and Owen 2008; McDonald 2012; Liminana-Gras et al. 2013; Ratcliff 2002).

## The influence of women within CIM use and practice

### Informal CIM care

Women are important sources of information and decision-making within the community not just for their own health care but also with regards to the care of others (including parents, children, spouses and extended family) (Cormac 2010; Dahlberg et al. 2007; George 2008; Weir 2005). Research suggests these circumstances also apply to CIM use with women not only identified as predominant users of CIM (Reid et al. 2017; Zhang et al. 2015) but also as significant agents of influence upon the CIM use of others – family members, friends and wider networks alike (Frawley et al. 2017; Murthy et al. 2017). The findings from such work suggest women have a significant role in the informal (and in the vast majority of cases hidden) provision and practice of CIM.

## *Formal CIM care*

Moving attention beyond informal care and carer roles, research has also suggested gender dimensions to CIM practice. For example, the increasing *mainstreaming* of CIM practices is arguably a gendered development. If we concentrate momentarily upon the growing trend by which some conventional medical and health care professions and personnel directly integrate aspects of CIM into conventional medical sites with no involvement of non-medical CIM providers – what some commentators have labelled direct integrative practice (Adams and Tovey 2000) – we see integration is often driven by those conventional health professions (nursing and midwifery, for example) (Adams and Tovey 2000; Boughn and Lentini 1999; Cant et al. 2011; Cant et al. 2012) that have female-dominated workforces (Allen 2004; Carpenter 1993; Manley 1995). Indeed, in some analyses, it has been suggested that a prime motivation for direct integrative practice may itself be closely connected to wider professional struggles that can be interpreted as partly products of the male domination of health care and models of delivery (see Adams 2006).

Focusing upon the direct ranks of the CIM workforce – the vast majority of which is located in private practice beyond regular, in-depth collaboration with conventional medical and health care professions – we can identify interesting gender patterns among practitioner groups. Given the exponential growth in popularity of CIM over recent decades, it is somewhat surprising that the CIM workforce has not received more research attention. Indeed, a review of the recent literature over the last decade reveals a dearth of in-depth, quality analysis relating to the ranks of the CIM workforce, a failing identified by previous authors (Nissen 2011; Stumpf et al. 2010) and which still remains.

Nevertheless, from the early ad-hoc work that has been undertaken on this topic we can at least identify some rudimentary descriptions of the CIM workforce pertaining to gender composition. Probably the most wide-ranging analysis on CIM workforce characteristics has been undertaken by Leach (2013). While acknowledging a number of important limitations to this work (Frawley 2016), this study, based upon relevant population census data, examined practitioner ranks across Australia, New Zealand, Canada, the United States and the United Kingdom to provide some initial insights. With regards to gender composition, this work identified practitioners as typically female across the broad CIM workforce (Leach 2013). However, upon closer analysis, Leach also identifies cross-country trends that can be interpreted as the basis of two *ideal-type* gender compositions with regards to different CIM practitioner ranks. First, are a number of CIM modalities that appear to be male-dominated (with a small number of country exceptions) which appear to be representative of chiropractic, osteopathy and acupuncture (ranging from just over half of all practitioners being male to roughly two male practitioners to every female practitioner) and acupuncture to a lesser extent. Meanwhile, this 2013 study found occupations such as massage therapy, naturopathy and homeopathy were female-dominated where there were at least three female practitioners to every male (ibid.).

Other literature on the gender composition in CIM workforce has tended to fall within these ideal-type generalizations with regards to herbalists (Leach et al. 2014), a range of CIM practitioners (Grace 2013), massage therapists (Smith et al. 2011; Wardle et al. 2015) and chiropractors (Adams et al. 2017). One interesting aspect of this ideal-type demarcation regarding gender composition within different CIM professions is how it relates to a number of broader more conceptually and theoretically-driven analyses and interpretations relating to gender, CIM practice and the potential of a feminist model of health and health care.

## CIM practice: a feminist model of health and care?

Moving beyond a descriptive account of the gender composition in CIM ranks has been a small body of research examining the relationship between gender and CIM practice (Flesch 2007, 2010; Nissen 2011; Scott 1998).[1] A number of writers have highlighted how women's CIM practice and use may shed light on or resonate with the feminist health project more generally (Nissen 2011; Scott 1998) constituting a potential site of resistance against the dominant biomedical model of health and health care. This is seen in terms of, among other things, recasting the nature of women's CIM practitioner-patient relationship as an egalitarian partnership (Nissen 2011) where women's experiences, distinct knowledges and personal ways of knowing are central to practice and women are empowered through their CIM use. Based upon a range of fieldwork experiences, including study of homeopaths (Scott 1998), students of acupuncture and oriental medicine (Flesch 2010) and herbalists (Barry 2003; Nissen 2008), it is purported that 'women's practice and use of CIM present an opportunity to fulfil and confront traditional gender roles and discourses of femininity' (Nissen 2011).

However, within and beyond this body of literature some writers have highlighted a number of potential developments relating to CIM that may challenge an ability to realize CIM practice as a feminist model of health care. For example, Flesch (2007) highlights how the professionalization process and gender are interwined. Professionalization – the process through which an occupation seeks state-sanctioned self-regulation, social closure and jurisdictional claims around 'turf' – has been of some success for CIM groups. Through this process, many CIM modalities have achieved greater state legitimacy (Almeida and Gabe 2016; Saks 2015) and statutory recognition in a number of jurisdictions (Baer 2003; Kelner et al. 2004: Kelner and Wellman 2006). Furthermore, as Flesch outlines, the biomedical path of professionalization has been the archetype for similar CIM advances in this area and, as she argues, such professionalization may itself deny 'both the unique philosophy of [CIM] and the existence of alternative, feminine conceptions of professionalism' (Flesch 2007: 168).

Similarly, a number of writers, including both Flesch (2007) and Turner (2004), highlight how different forms of CIM co-opting as found in contemporary health care may lead to sacrificing core tenets of CIM (central to the feminist model of care), such as holism, women's empowerment and the democratization of knowledge. Flesch (2007) is focused upon how conventional medicine's more recent cautious acceptance of CIM is predicated upon CIM being evaluated via the same standards of evidence as biomedicine and CIM education incorporating increased biomedical knowledge content. Meanwhile, Turner (2004) is more interested in how the move towards CIM integration within conventional settings and dominant socio-political systems may co-opt a number of fringe and radical meanings and ways of knowing/doing, resulting in CIM comfortably sitting within the dominant biomedical paradigm of health. Drawing upon different circumstances around CIM growth in modern health systems, Collyer (2004) also highlights how the increasing corporatization and commercialization of CIM, what she sees as a part of *mainstreaming*, have led to decreased autonomy among CIM practitioners with increasing numbers finding themselves 'employed by corporations such as vitamin or pharmaceutical companies [and] in corporately owned "integrated" or "holistic" clinics' (Collyer 2004: 88–89). Equally, the recent boom in retail outlets and pharmacy to stock over-the-counter supplements and natural products also creates further disconnect between CIM and wider philosophy or consultation styles.

## Conclusion

As identified in the brief overview provided in this chapter, the influence and role of women with regards to CIM provision/workforce, practice and consumption are considerable. Indeed, while CIM is quite obviously applicable across gender, women have played and continue to play a crucial role in the growth and sustainability of CIM with regards to both the informal and formal health care arenas. The extent to which CIM practices (all or a selection) are themselves (to varying degrees) feminist or gendered forms of health care and practice remains contested in the face of globalization, mass markets, the rise of corporatism and commercialization and the increasing push for legitimacy and professionalization of the wider CIM project. Similarly, with the growing calls for CIM to adopt the standards of evidence-based medicine and the gold standard clinical trial design (Ernst 2002; Pirotta 2007), notwithstanding what many have outlined as complex and in some ways inadequate designs for CIM (Verhoef et al. 2005; Verhoef and Vanderhayden 2007), it would appear that some of the more radical possibilities of CIM practice for the feminist project may fail to be (widely) realized.

What does remain, however, is the major role CIM continues to play as a highly positive influence on the health and life of women with regards to their own health and that of others in their familial and community networks and with regards to their commitment and role in formal health care practice and delivery. It is striking that the last decade shows only marginal research interest in the gendered aspects of CIM and the contemporary environment of health practice and systems appears to continue to uphold key aspects of the dominant biomedical model of care. Whether future years will continue to pose challenges to frustrate the potential of CIM to radically reshape and redefine the nature and approach to health and health care that reflects women's perspectives, experiences and needs remains to be seen but as the wider history of professional struggle with regards to women and health care shows, the dominant paradigm of health and the power of the male-dominated professional project are unlikely to quickly concede ground to new and opposing interests. It remains that the in-depth examination of the relationship between gender and CIM practice is a broad topic worthy of future attention and holding much potential to provide rich insights regarding the current and future role of CIM within health systems and wider culture.

## Note

1   In this chapter we focus upon the CIM workforce located in private practice beyond conventional medicine and personnel, but it is worth noting that interesting work has been done examining the extent and ways in which the rhetoric of integrative medicine and integrative medical practitioners in the USA can be interpreted as performing a feminist intervention in biomedical discourse and may hold the potential to significantly reframe health care practices in conventional clinical sites (Willard 2005).

## References

Abbott, A. (1988) *The System of Professions: An Essay on the Division of Labour*, Chicago: University of Chicago Press.

Adams, J. (2006) 'An exploratory study of complemntary and alternative medicine in hospital midwifery: models of care and professional struggle', *Complementary Therapies in Clinical Practice*, 12(1): 40–47.

Adams, J., Lauche, R., Peng, W. et al. (2017) 'A workforce survey of Australian chiropractic: the profile and practice features of a nationally representative sample of 2,005 chiropractors', *BMC Complementary and Alternative Medicine*, 17: 14.

Adams, J. and Tovey, P. (2000) 'Complementary medicine and primary care: towards a grassroots focus', in P. Tovey (ed.) *Contemporary Primary Care: The Challenges of Change*, Buckingham: Open University Press.

AIHW (Australian Institute of Health and Welfare) (2012) *Medical Practitioners Workforce 2012*. Available at: www.aihw.gov.au/reports/workforce-2012

AIHW (Australian Institute of Health and Welfare) (2013) *Medical Practitioners Workforce 2013*. Available at: www.aihw.gov.au/reports/workforce-2013

AIHW (Australian Institute of Health and Welfare) (2014) *Medical Practitioners Workforce 2014*. Available at: www.aihw.gov.au/reports/workforce-2014

AIHW (Australian Institute of Health and Welfare) (2016) *Medical Practitioners Workforce 2016*. Available at: www.aihw.gov.au/reports/workforce-2016

Allen, D. (2004) 'The nursing-medical boundary: a negotiated order?', in E. Annanndale, M. Elston and L. Prior (eds) *Medical Work, Medical Knowledge and Health Care*, Oxford: Blackwell.

Almeida, J. and Gabe, J. (2016) 'CAM within a field force of countervailing powers: the case of Portugal', *Social Science and Medicine*, 155: 73–81.

Baer, H. (2006) 'The drive for legitimation in Australian naturopathy: successes and dilemmas', *Social Science and Medicine*, 63: 1771–1783.

Barry, C. A. (2003) 'The body, health, and healing in alternative and integrated medicine: An ethnography of homeopathy in South London', unpublished PhD thesis, Brunel University.

Boughn, S. and Lentini, A. (1999) 'Why do women choose nursing?', *Journal of Nursing Education*, 38(4): 156–161.

Cant, S., Watts, P. and Ruston, A. (2011) 'Negotiating competency, professionalism and risk: the integration of complementary and alternative medicine by nurses and midwives in NHS hospitals', *Social Science and Medicine*, 72: 529–536.

Cant, S., Watts, P. and Ruston, A. (2012) 'The rise and fall of complementary medicine in National Health Service hospitals in England', *Social Science and Medicine*, 18: 135–139.

Carpenter, M. (1993) 'The subordination of nurses in health care: towards a social divisions approach', in E. Riska and K. Wegar (eds) *Gender, Work and Medicine: Women and the Medical Division of Labour*, London: Sage.

Collyer, F. (2004) 'The corporatisation and commercialisation of CAM', in P. Tovey, G. Easthope and J. Adams (eds) *The Mainstreaming of Complementary and Alternative Medicine: Studies in Social Context*, London: Routledge.

Cormac, I. (2010) 'Women as carers', in D. Kohen (ed.) *Oxford Textbook of Women and Mental Health*, Oxford: Oxford University Press.

Dahlberg, L., Demack, S., Bambra, C. (2007) 'Age and gender of informal carers: a population-based study in the UK', *Health and Social Care in the Community*, 15(5): 439–445.

Doel, M. and Segrott, J. (2003) 'Self, health, and gender: complementary and alternative medicine in the British mass media', *Gender, Place and Culture: A Journal of Feminist Geography*, 10(2): 131–144.

Ernst, E. (2002) 'What's the point of rigorous research on complementary/alternative medicine?', *Journal of the Royal Society of Medicine*, 95(4): 211–213.

Flesch, H. (2007) 'Silent voices: women, complementary medicine, and the co-optation of change', *Complementary Therapies in Clinical Practice*, 13(3): 166–173.

Flesch, H. (2010) 'Balancing act: women and the study of complementary and alternative medicine', *Complementary Therapies in Clinical Practice*, 16: 20–25.

Frawley, J. E. (2016) 'Complementary and alternative medicine in Australia: an overview of contemporary workforce features'. *Australian Journal of Herbal Medicine*, 28(4): 103–105.

Frawley, J., Anheyer, D., Davidson, S. and Jackson, D. (2017) 'Prevalence and characteristics of complementary and alternative medicine use by Australian children', *Journal of Paediatrics and Child Health*, 53: 782–787.

Friedson, E. (1970) *Profession of Medicine: A Study of the Sociology of Applied Knowledge*, New York: Dodd, Mead and Company.

George, A. (2008) 'Nurses, communtiy health workers, and home carers: gendered human resources compensating for skewed health systems', *Global Public Health*, 3(S1): 75–89.

Gjerberg, E. (2001) 'Medical women – towards full integration? An analysis of the specialty choices made by two cohorts of Norwegian doctors', *Social Science and Medicine*, 52: 331–343.

Goldner, M. (2004) 'Consumption as activism: an examination of CAM as part of the consumer movement in health', in P. Tovey, G. Easthope and J. Adams (eds) *The*

*Mainstreaming of Complementary and Alternative Medicine: Studies in Social Context*, London: Routledge.

Grace, S. (2012) 'CAM practitioners in the Australian health workforce: an underutilized resource', *BMC Complementary and Alternative Medicine*, 12: 205.

Hammond, J. (2009) 'Assessment of clinical components of physiotherapy undergraduate education: are there any issues with gender?', *Physiotherapy*, 95(4): 266–272.

Heiligers, P. and Hingstman, L. (2000) 'Career preferences and work-family balance in medicine: gender differences among medical specialists', *Social Science and Medicine*, 50: 1235–1246.

Hojat, M., Gonnella, J. and Erdmann, J. (2000) 'Physicians' perceptions of the changing health care system: comparisons by gender and specialties', *Journal of Community Health*, 25(6): 455–471.

Inhorn, M. and Whittle, K. (2001) 'Feminism meets the "new" epidemiologies: towards an appraisal of antifeminist biases in epidemiological research on women's health', *Social Science and Medicine*, 53: 553–567.

Kell, C. and Owen, G. (2008) 'Physiotherapy as a profession: where are we now?', *International Journal of Therapy and Rehabilitation*, 15(4): 158–164.

Kelner, M., Wellman, B., Boon, H. and Welsh, S. (2004) 'Responses of established healthcare to the professionalization of complementary and alternative medicine in Ontario', *Social Science and Medicine*, 59: 915–930.

Kelner, M. and Wellman, B. (2006) 'How far can complementary and alternative medicine go? The case of chiropractic and homeopathy', *Social Science and Medicine*, 63: 2617–2627.

Kilminster, S., Downes, J., Gough, B., Murdoch-Eaton, D. and Roberts, T, (2007) 'Women in medicine – is there a problem? A literature review of the changing gender composition, structures and occupational cultures in medicine', *Medical Education*, 41(1): 39–49.

Leach, M. (2013) 'Profile of the complementary and alternative medicine workforce across Australia, New Zealand, Canada, United States and United Kingdom', *Complementary Therapies in Medicine*, 21: 364–378.

Leach, M., McIntyre, E. and Frawley, J. (2014) 'Characteristics of the Australian complementary and alternative medicine (CAM) workforce', *Australian Journal of Herbal Medicine*, 26(2): 58–65.

Levinson, W. and Lurie, N. (2004) 'When most doctors are women: what lies ahead?' *Annals of Internal Medicine*, 141(6), 471–474.

Liminana-Gras, R., Sanchez-Lopez, M., Roman, A. and Corbala-Berna, F. (2013) 'Health and gender in female-dominated occupations: the case of male nurses', *The Journal of Men's Studies*, 21(2): 135–148.

Manley, J. (1995) 'Sex-segregated work in the system of professions: the development and stratification in nursing', *Sociological Quarterly*, 36: 297–314.

McDonald, J. (2012) 'Conforming to and resisting dominant gender norms: how male and female nursing students do and undo gender', *Gender, Work and Organisation*, 20(5): 561–579.

Murthy, V., Adams, J., Broom, A. et al. (2017) 'The influence of communication and information sources upon decision-making around complementary and alternative medicine use for back pain amongst Australian women aged 60–65 years', *Health and Social Care in the Community*, 25(1): 114–122.

Nissen N. (2008) 'Herbal healthcare and processes of change: an ethnographic study of women's contemporary practice and use of Western herbal medicine in the UK, unpublished PhD thesis, The Open University.

Nissen, N. (2011) 'Challenging perspectives: women, complementary and alternative medicine, and social change', *Interface: A Journal for and about Social Movements*, 3: 187–212.

Pirotta, M. (2007) 'Towards the application of RCTs for CAM', in J. Adams (ed.) *Researching Complementary and Alternative Medicine*, London: Routledge.

Ratcliff, K. (2002) *Women and Health: Power, Technology, Inequality and Conflict in a Gendered World*, Boston: Allyn and Bacon.

Reid, R. (2017) 'The traditional naturopathic treatments utilised for the management of endometriosis and associated symptoms,' *Australian Journal of Herbal Medicine*, *29*(1): 38–39.

Reid, R., Steel, A., Wardle, J., Trubody, A. and Adams, J. (2016) 'Complementary medicine use by the Australian population: a critical mixed studies systematic review of utilisation, perceptions and factors associated with use', *BMC Complementary and Alternative Medicine*, 16: 176.

Riska, E. (2001) 'Towards gender balance: but will women physicians have an impact on medicine?', *Social Science and Medicine*, 52: 179–187.

Riska, E. and Wegar, K. (eds) (1993) *Gender, Work and Medicine: Women and the Medical Division of Labour*, London: Sage.Rogers, W. (2004) 'Evidence-based medicine and women: do the principles and practice of EBM further women's health?', *Bioethics*, 18(1): 50–71.

Saks, M. (2015) *The Professions, State and the Market: Medicine in Britain, the United States and Russia*, New York: Routledge.

Schiebinger, L. (2003) 'Women's health and clinical trials', *The Journal of Clinical Investigation*,112(7): 973–977.

Scott, A. L. (1998) 'The symbolizing body and the metaphysics of alternative medicine', *Body & Society*, 4(3): 21–37.

Smith, J., Sullivan, S. and Baxter, G. (2011) 'A descriptive study of the practice patterns of New Zealand massage therapists', *International Journal of Therapeutic Massage and Bodywork*, 4(1): 18–27.

Smith-Cunnien, S. (1998) *A Profession of One's Own: Organised Medicine's Opposition to Chiropractic*, New York: University Press of America.

Stumpf, S., Hardy, M., Kendall, D. and Carr, C. (2010) 'Unveiling the United States acupuncture workforce', *Complementary Health Practice Review*, 15(1): 31–39.

Turner, P. K. (2004) 'Mainstreaming alternative medicine: doing midwifery at the intersection', *Qualitative Health Research*, 14*(*5): 644–662.

Verhoef, M., Lewith, G., Ritenbaugh, C. et al.(2005) 'CAM whole systems research: beyond identifying the inadequacies of the RCT', *Complementary Therapies in Medicine*, 13(3): 2006–2012.

Verhoef, M. and Vanderhayden, L. (2007) 'Combining qualitative methods and RCTs in CAM intervention research', in J. Adams (ed.) *Researching Complementary and Alternative Medicine*, London: Routledge.

Wardle, J. and Adams, J. (2012) 'Naturopaths: their role in primary health care delivery', in J. Adams, P. Magin and A. Broom (eds) *Primary Health Care and complementary and Integrative Medicine: Practice and Research*, London: Imperial College Press.

Wardle, J., Barnett, R. and Adams, J. (2015) 'Practice and research in Australian massage therapy: a national workforce survey', *International Journal of Therapeutic Massage and Bodywork*, 8(2): 2–11.

Weir, A. (2005) 'The global universal caregiver: imagining women's liberation in the new millennium', *Constellations*, 12(3): 308–330.

Welsh, S., Kelner, M., Wellman, B. and Boon, H. (2004) 'Moving forward? Complementary and alternative practitioners seeking self-regulation', *Sociology of Health & Illness*, 26(2): 216–241.

Willard, B. (2005) 'Feminist interventions in biomedical discourse: an analysis of the rhetoric of integrative medicine', *Women's Studies in Communication*, 28(1): 115–148.

Zhang, Y., Leach, M., Hall, H., et al. (2015) 'Differences between male and female consumption of complementary and alternative medicine in a national US population: a secondary analysis of 2012 NHIS data', *Evidence-Based Complementary and Alternative Medicine*, doi:10.1155/2015/413173.

# 11 Models of care and women's health

## Drawing upon aspects of complementary and integrative medicine

*Matthew Leach, Amie Steel and Jon Adams*

### Introduction

A lack of availability and accessibility of health care services and satisfaction of health care services are all cited as contributing to women frequently reporting high levels of unmet health care need (Pappa et al. 2013). In fact, many women appear dissatisfied with conventional medicine and are turning to other services such as complementary and integrative medicine (CIM) (Steel et al. 2012). This suggests that conventional health care systems may be failing to adequately meet the needs of women, and that other health services and perhaps different models of care may have the potential to play an important role in addressing this challenge.

A model of care – 'overarching design for the provision of a particular type of health care service that is shaped by a theoretical basis, evidence-based practice, and defined standards' (Davidson et al. 2006) – determines the manner through which health services are delivered by outlining best practice care and services for a person, population group or patient cohort as they progress through the stages of a condition, injury or event (ACI 2013). In this chapter, we aim to describe the disconnect between women's health care needs and the dominant model of health care, and explore the role CIM can, and in some cases already does, play in addressing women's unmet health care needs.

In the first section of this chapter, we explore these needs from a historical perspective describing the way women's health has been understood and managed in the past, and how this has been shaped by a woman's position in society at different times. The chapter then proceeds to look at the components that define a high-quality health care system by drawing upon the key dimensions of health care system performance. These dimensions will be used to create a set of minimum standards necessary to achieve a woman-centred model of care. The penultimate section of the chapter examines the model of health – the biomedical model – currently dominating clinical decision making in most health systems across the globe. In light of the limitations of the biomedical model, a new model of care is proposed to address the biopsychosocial needs of women. The model draws from the strengths of the biomedical model, as well as other models of care (e.g. CIM systems), to create a comprehensive, holistic and women-centred model of care that meets the standards expected of a high-performing, contemporary health care service.

## The health care needs of women

The health care needs of women were largely ignored up until the late twentieth century and up until this time, many women's health complaints were ascribed to demonic possession, hysteria, hypochondria and witchcraft (Tasca et al. 2012). While the modern era has shed new light on the aetiology of many reproductive, sexual and mental disorders, the twenty-first century has also seen the rise of a range of new concerns around the health of women, including female sexual dysfunction (Hayes et al. 2008), eating disorders (Duncan, Ziobrowski and Nicol 2017) and body image issues (Petroski, Pelegrini and Glaner 2012). Adding to this are emerging concerns regarding sex differences in the aetiology, diagnosis and management of health disorders (Kautzky-Willer and Harreiter 2017), which not only highlight women's health care needs as distinct from those of men, but also that diagnosis and management of these disorders requires a gender-specific approach.

Socio-political drivers over the past few decades (e.g. the women's health movement) have secured women's health on national and international policy agendas and empowered women to regain control of their health (Morgen 2002). This has resulted in progress such as the implementation of national cervical cancer screening programmes (Saville 2015), breast cancer screening programmes (Lauby-Secretan et al. 2015) and preconception care programmes (Steel et al. 2016). Nevertheless, the actual needs and preferences of women in terms of the models through which these services are delivered have not been given close research attention (ibid.), and as such, there is still much more to be done to adequately address the plethora of women's health care needs in contemporary health systems.

## Indicators of a high-quality health care system

Health care systems have transformed considerably over the past century. One major change has been the shift away from institutionalised to community-based care (Baldwin 1993; Shen and Snowden 2014). in part, driven by a need to reduce the stigma of disease, to foster individual autonomy and patient empowerment (Shen and Snowden 2014), and to reduce health care costs (Baldwin 1993). As well as transformations in the bricks and mortar of health care delivery, the past few decades have witnessed considerable changes in models of care, health technology and our understanding of the aetiology and management of human disease. While these changes may be viewed as 'advances' in health care, the question remains: do these changes and contemporary circumstances reflect and address the health care needs of the (female) population? In order to answer this question, it is important to first understand the elements that define a high-quality health care system.

Health care performance indicators, used by many countries as a means of evaluating the quality of a health care system, are typically organised around dimensions of performance. A recent review highlights the dimensions of performance indicator frameworks used in eight Organisation for Economic Co-operation and Development (OECD) countries (Braithwaite et al. 2017). The review found 401 nationally consistent and locally relevant indicators of health service performance, which were best represented by the following five dimensions: (1) patient experience; (2) efficiency; (3) safety and quality; (4) population health outcomes; and (5) access.

- The first dimension, *patient experience*, encompasses several different constructs, including satisfaction with care, individualised care and patient-centred care (Wolf et al. 2014). Satisfaction with care also comprises many elements, but the most consistent determinants of satisfaction are provider-related factors, including courtesy, empathy, respect, careful listening, communication, and regard for patient preference (Al-Abri and Al-Balushi 2014). Related to satisfaction with care is the issue of choice; this refers to the extent to which a system enables patients to select the provider, treatment, institution or insurer of their choosing. As for the constructs of individualised care and patient-centred care, these terms are often used interchangeably, albeit incorrectly; the former referring to the tailoring of care to a patient's unique experiences, feelings and behaviours (Radwin and Alster 2002), and the latter relating to a therapeutic partnership in which a patient's needs, preferences and goals are prioritised (Epstein and Street 2011). Although many of the elements that fall under the experience dimension are also captured within national charters/bills of patient rights (American Hospital Association 2003; Australian Commission on Safety and Quality in Health Care 2009; Williams 2015), individualised care and patient-centred receive little recognition in these charters/bills.
- The second dimension, *efficiency*, refers to the appropriate allocation of resources, setting of priorities, adaptability to change, and effective outcomes of care (Duckett 1999). Embedded within this dimension are many different constructs, including evidence-based practice, economic evaluation, resource allocation, access, quality and safety. It is important to note that efficiency is not just the responsibility of government and administrators; it is a matter requiring the involvement of all stakeholders, including patients (e.g. adherence to treatment), providers (e.g. adherence to evidence-based clinical guidelines), communities (e.g. using appropriate patient monitoring/tracking systems), and health services (e.g. using appropriate models of care) (Smith 2012). In simple terms, efficiency is about getting the right staff/skill mix/services to the right place at the right time at the right cost in order to achieve the right outcomes.

- *Safety and quality* represent the third dimension of health care performance. Quality itself is not easily defined, but an earlier definition by the Institute of Medicine seems to provide some clarity, referring to quality as 'the degree to which health services for individuals and populations increase the likelihood of desired health outcomes and are consistent with current professional knowledge' (Lohr 1990). Safety, an integral component of quality, is concerned with minimising the incidence and impact of, and maximising recovery from, adverse events (Emanuel et al. 2008). Put simply, quality and safety are about achieving optimal health outcomes for individuals with the least risk of harm.

- *Population health outcomes* are the fourth dimension of health care performance. This dimension refers to the health status of the population, rather than its individual members, which is helpful in understanding the collective impact of a health care system (Stoto 2014). Importantly, a population health perspective looks beyond the health system, and takes into account the influence of other important social and environmental determinants of health, such as policy, law, family, community, water supply, air quality, and built and natural environments (Teutsch, Herman and Teutsch 2016). Further, relative to the disease-centred focus of mainstream health care, population health has a strong focus on health promotion, disease prevention and quality of life (Parrish 2010). Thus, implicit in the dimension of population health are the constructs of holism, well-being and prevention, which align not only with an ecologic model of health (Teutsch, Herman and Teutsch 2016), but also the core principles of CIM (Leach 2010).

- The final dimension of health care performance, *access*, refers to 'the opportunity to identify health care needs, to seek healthcare services, to reach, to obtain or use healthcare services and to actually have the need for services fulfilled' (Levesque, Harris and Russell 2013). Thus, access ensures that factors affecting one's ability to perceive (e.g. health literacy, health beliefs), seek (e.g. gender, culture), reach (e.g. transport, mobility), pay (e.g. income, health insurance) or engage (e.g. empowerment, information) with the health care system do not discriminate a person from receiving needed or desired services (ibid.).

While it is acknowledged that a health care system cannot be all things to all people, it should at least go some way towards addressing the health needs of the population (Wilson-Stronks et al. 2008). The provision of a health care system that focuses solely on patient experience, efficiency, safety and quality, population health outcomes and access, in a literal sense, is unlikely to be enough to serve the distinct needs of individuals in a given population (Rouse 2008). However, if the system also incorporates many implicit constructs of these dimensions, such as individualised care, patient-centredness, holism, evidence-based practice, well-being and prevention, then it will be more attuned to addressing individuals' health needs.

*Strengths and limitations of biomedicine*

Most contemporary health care systems are underpinned by a biomedical model of care; embracing a mechanistic view, perceiving the mind and body as separate entities, and focusing on affective, physiological therapeutic interventions while largely disregarding an individual's psychosocial factors (Cantor 2003). While biomedicine has undoubtedly enabled significant advances in the science of treating disease and has provided an essential platform for supporting improved efficiency in health care delivery and patient outcomes (Worrall, Chaulk and Freake 1997), the biomedical model has encouraged clinical care that largely disregards the complexities of the individual patients' psychological, spiritual, and social life as it relates to their health (Hewa and Hetherington 1995).

In the context of women's health, the biomedical model has afforded advances in the diagnosis and treatment of women's health complaints (Bentivegna et al. 2016), yet the dehumanised approach of the biomedical model often results in medical practitioners providing care inadequate to the health care needs of women (Steel et al. 2016). While the 'endemic dehumanisation' of biomedicine has a functional benefit in some instances, such as improved capacity for doctors to problem solve and regulate negative emotions in the face of trauma and high stress clinical environments, this approach has been juxtaposed by scholars advocating the need for a greater focus on person-centred medicine, of which CIM should play a fundamental role (di Sarsina, Alivia and Guadagni 2013).

## A proposed model of care for women's health with a focus upon CIM

Given the limitations of the biomedical model of care, it appears that this model may well face challenges in addressing the distinct health care needs of women. Consequently, there is a need to rethink how health care is delivered to women so that the health care needs of this population do not remain unmet. Outlined below are the *twelve objectives* (grouped around broader themes of patient experience, efficiency, population health outcomes, access, safety and quality) of an ideal model of care for women's health.

*Patient experience*

*   *Patient satisfaction* impacts treatment adherence, health outcomes and engage-ment in preventive care (Doyle, Lennox and Bell 2013), and is a valuable proxy indicator of the quality of clinician and health service performance (Prakash 2010). In the context of women's health, satisfaction with care should be considered in the management of health conditions both unique to women (such as pregnancy and childbirth or menstrual disorders) (Hodnett 2002) and those affecting the wider population but where women's satisfaction with care may differ from men (Kressin et al. 1999). It is also important that clinicians and health services identify issues that impact a women's satisfaction with health care as they arise, and promptly take steps to remedy these issues.

- *Patient choice* is positively correlated with patient satisfaction (Costa-Font and Zigante 2016), which can empower individuals and strengthen the therapeutic relationship (Tynkkynen et al. 2016). At a health system level, increasing health care choice may help incentivise providers to improve the quality and efficiency of services (Costa-Font and Zigante 2016). Despite the acknowledged value in respecting patient choice, women still perceive a lack of support for their preferences in many aspects of contemporary health care provision (Nieuwenhuijze and Low 2013). Meanwhile, CIM is commonly described by women as empowering and supportive of individual choice (Nissen 2011); hence, CIM may be considered a fundamental component of a model of care for women's health.

- *Individualised care* is associated with improvements in patient satisfaction and well-being (Rathert, Wyrwich and Boren 2012) and is an acknowledged feature of CIM (Franzel et al. 2013). In line with the principles of individualised care, clinicians should tailor the plan of care, wherever possible, to the patient's unique experiences, feelings and behaviours (Radwin and Alster 2002). Characteristics that women may bring to a health care encounter, which would require an individualised approach, would include ethnicity (Pavlish, Noor and Brandt 2010), religion (Hasnain et al. 2011), and history of trauma (Wilson 2010), among others.

- *Patient-centred care* may contribute to improvements in patient outcomes, including patient well-being and satisfaction, as well as patient mortality and disability (Olsson et al. 2013). To enhance the patient experience, clinicians should foster a therapeutic partnership that prioritises a patient's needs, preferences and goals (Epstein and Street 2011). Structural factors are also paramount, which should take into account the patient-centredness of the health care environment and administrative processes (Greene, Tuzzio and Cherkin 2012); an approach increasingly acknowledged in aspects of women's health, such as maternity care (Shaw et al. 2016), and reported to be experienced by individuals accessing care from a CIM practitioner (Foley and Steel 2017b).

## Efficiency

- *Evidence-based care* is shown to be associated with better patient outcomes, reduced health care costs and shorter lengths of stay when compared with standard care (Emparanza, Cabello and Burls 2015). Clinicians should therefore ensure that clinical decisions are informed by the best available evidence, in conjunction with clinical expertise, patient preference and resource availability. Health services should support the implementation of evidence-based practice (EBP) by improving clinician skills and access to evidence-based resources, and embracing a culture of EBP (Leach and Tucker 2017a; 2017b). The degree to which CIM can address this dimension within the context of women's health is unclear as both the evidence base for CIM practices and the degree to which evidence informs clinical decision-making for CIM practitioners are variable at best (Leach and Gillham 2011).

- *Economic evaluation* assists in promoting the delivery of a more efficient health system/model of care by prioritising interventions that represent a more effective use of resources amidst multiple competing options (Dang, Likhar and Alok 2016). Clinicians should be aware of the economic impact of various treatment options – for the institution, the health care system and the individual patient – and should give this due consideration when formulating a plan of care with the patient and significant others. Emerging evidence suggests CIM may be cost-effective and contribute to possible cost savings in some clinical populations, including pregnant women and older women experiencing low back pain (Herman et al. 2012).

- *Resource allocation* within the context of a health care setting (as opposed to a health care system) refers to the rationing of health care resources to different patients or patient groups (Angelis, Kanavos and Montibeller 2017). To facilitate the efficiency of a women-centred model of care, clinicians should ensure clinical decisions are fair, legitimate and transparent, are based on relevant reasoning, and are responsive to a changing evidence base (ibid.). Thus, where sufficient evidence of safety and effectiveness emerges for an intervention (including a CIM treatment), particularly if it is shown to address an unmet health care need (such as acupuncture for primary dysmenorrhoea) (Abaraogu and Tabansi-Ochuogu 2015), resources should be allocated to support its inclusion in health care settings that adopt a women-centred model of care.

## Population health outcomes

- *Holism* – the intentional consideration of bio-psycho-sociocultural factors in all aspects of a patient's care – has been shown to be related to improvements in patient satisfaction (Esch et al. 2008). A holistic approach is also an important prerequisite for delivering individualised care (Demirsoy 2017), is strongly associated with CIM (Foley and Steel 2017a) and shares many characteristics with the patient-centred care movement (Foley and Steel 2017b). Further, the absence of holism in contemporary health care has been noted as an important push factor for women choosing to access CIM (Meurk et al. 2013). Accordingly, clinicians should ensure that biological, psychological, spiritual, cultural and environmental factors are taken into account in the diagnosis, planning, implementation and evaluation of a woman's care.

- *Well-being* represents a multi-dimensional construct of social, physical and psychological function and health (Pressman, Kraft and Bowlin 2013). Evidence indicates that patient well-being may be positively associated with patient satisfaction (Clement and Burnett 2013), and that staff well-being is an important antecedent to patient well-being (Maben 2014). Thus, not only should clinicians evaluate patients' well-being and put in place strategies to improve a patient's social, physical and psychological function, but so should health services (for staff). CIM appears to have a fundamental role in improving and maintaining individual well-being (WHO 2013), and is an important reason why many women use CIM (Gollschewski et al. 2008) and why CIM should be an integral component of a women-centred model of care.

• *Prevention*, particularly the provision of evidence-based preventive services and screening, may contribute to better patient outcomes and improvements in health system efficiency (Maciosek et al. 2010). Consequently, clinicians should ensure patient care plans incorporate primary/secondary/tertiary prevention strategies, where appropriate. Similarly, health services should invest in appropriate infrastructure (e.g. personnel) to support the provision of preventive services and screening. Many systems of medicine within the broad remit of CIM embrace the principles of prevention (Foley and Steel 2017c), with evidence suggesting that CIM practitioners are now playing a more active role in preventive women's health, such as preconception care (Steel et al. 2017).

## Access

*Access* relates to a person's ability to *perceive* (e.g. level of health literacy), *seek* (e.g. availability of female health providers), *reach* (e.g. accessibility of transportation), *pay* (e.g. level of disposable personal income) or *engage* (e.g. level of information) with the health care system (Levesque, Harris and Russell 2013). Reduced access to health care services is associated with poorer health outcomes (Puthussery 2016), thus health services should ensure appropriate infrastructure, staffing and financing options to mitigate potential barriers to health care access. The provision of CIM services may be seen to facilitate a women's access to health care in some regards, for example, higher numbers of CIM practitioners in rural areas (Wardle, Lui and Adams 2012) or increased proportion of female CIM practitioners (Leach 2013). However, CIM may be considered a barrier to health care access in other ways (e.g. out-of-pocket costs) (Desai et al. 2013).

## Safety and quality

Safety and quality refer to the delivery of optimal health outcomes with minimal risk of adverse events; ensuring that benefits far outweigh any risk of harm to the patient, where appropriate. To achieve this goal, clinicians and health services should provide safe, effective, efficient, equitable, patient-centred and timely health care to all patients. Indeed, many CIM interventions have been identified as safer and as effective as relevant conventional medicines, such as St. John's wort for major depression (Linde, Berner and Kriston 2008) and garlic for dyslipidaemia (Ried, Toben and Fakler 2014). A women-centred model of care, which prioritises treatments demonstrating low risk of adverse events and convincing evidence of effectiveness, would be seen to meet this objective.

Translating these twelve objectives into a pragmatic model of care is an important next step. The six constructs of the chronic care model provide a useful framework through which to operationalise this proposed model of care for women's health. These constructs include the provision of organisational support, clinical information systems, delivery system design, decision support, self-management support, and community resources (Fiandt 2006). Emerging from the amalgamation of the above-mentioned objectives and the constructs of the chronic care model would be a model of care for women's health that not only addresses all modifiable components of health care delivery, but adequately serves the health care needs of women in contemporary society. Given that the dominant (biomedical) model of care has been largely inadequate in addressing the bio-psycho-sociocultural needs of women to date, the inclusion of CIM services is arguably an essential component of such a model, and would go some way towards supporting and manifesting the objectives of a high-quality health care service meeting the needs of women.

## Conclusion

Contemporary health policy acknowledges that an effective health care system provides models of care that not only support the health outcomes of the population but also deliver appropriate, accessible health care services that meet the needs of consumers; this includes the development of models of care that respond to the unique health care needs of women. The apparent disconnect between these needs and the features of contemporary health care may, in part, be remedied by more effective inclusion of CIM in the health system by offering women access to holistic, individualised and patient-centred care.

## References

Abaraogu, U. O. and Tabansi-Ochuogu, C. S. (2015) 'As acupressure decreases pain, acupuncture may improve some aspects of quality of life for women with primary dysmenorrhea: a systematic review with meta-analysis', *Journal of Acupuncture and Meridian Studies*, 8(5): 220–228.

Agency for Clinical Innovation (ACI) (2013) *Understanding the Process to Develop a Model of Care: An ACI Framework*, Chatswood, Australia: NSW Agency for Clinical Innovation.

Al-Abri, R. and Al-Balushi, A. (2014) 'Patient satisfaction survey as a tool towards quality improvement', *Oman Medical Journal*, 29(1): 3–7.

American Hospital Association (2003) *The Patient Care Partnership: Understanding Expectations, Rights and Responsibilities*, Atlanta, GA: American Hospital Association.

Angelis, A., Kanavos, P. and Montibeller, G. (2017) 'Resource allocation and priority setting in health care: a multi-criteria decision analysis problem of value?', *Global Policy*, 8(S2): 76–83.

Australian Commission on Safety and Quality in Health Care (ACSQHC) (2009) *About the Australian Charter of Healthcare Rights: A Guide for Healthcare Providers*. Sydney, Australia: ACSQHC.

Baldwin, S. (1993) *The Myth of Community Care: An Alternative Neighbourhood Model of Care*, Dordrecht: Springer Science and Business Media.

Bentivegna, E., Gouy, S., Maulard, A. et al. (2016) 'Oncological outcomes after fertility-sparing surgery for cervical cancer: a systematic review', *Lancet Oncology*, 17(6): e240–e253.

Braithwaite, J., Hibbert, P., Blakely, B. et al. (2017) 'Health system frameworks and performance indicators in eight countries: a comparative international analysis', *SAGE Open Medicine*, 5: 2050312116686516.

Cantor, D. (2003) 'The diseased body', in R. Cooter and J. Pickstone (eds) *A Companion to Medicine in the Twentieth Century*, London: Routledge.

Clement, N. D. and Burnett, R. (2013) 'Patient satisfaction after total knee arthroplasty is affected by their general physical well-being', *Knee Surgery, Sports Traumatology, Arthroscopy*, 21(11): 2638–2646.

Costa-Font, J. and Zigante, V. (2016) 'The choice agenda in European health systems: the role of middle-class demands', *Public Money Management*, 32(6): 409–416.

Dang, A., Likhar, N. and Alok, U. (2016) 'Importance of economic evaluation in health care: an Indian perspective', *Value and Health Regional Issues*, 9: 78–83.

Davidson, P., Halcomb, E., Hickman, L., Phillips, J. and Graham, B. (2006) 'Beyond the rhetoric: what do we mean by a "model of care"?', *Australian Journal of Advanced Nursing*, 23(3): 47–55.

Demirsoy, N. (2017) 'Holistic care philosophy for patient-centered approaches and spirituality', in O. Sayligil (ed.) *Patient-Centred Medicine*, Rijeka: In Tech Publishing.

Desai, M., Spelde, A., Knowlton, S. and Nava, A. (2013) 'Complementary and alternative medicine use, effectiveness, interest, and barriers to use at a tertiary-care pain medicine center', paper presented at the American Academy of Pain Medicine Annual Meeting, Fort Lauderdale, FL, April 11–14, 2013.

di Sarsina, P. R., Alivia, M. and Guadagni, P. (2013) 'The contribution of traditional, complementary and alternative medical systems to the development of person-centred medicine: the example of the charity association for person-centred medicine', *OA Alternative Medicine*, 1(2): 13.

Doyle, C., Lennox, L. and Bell, D. (2013) 'A systematic review of evidence on the links between patient experience and clinical safety and effectiveness', *BMJ Open*, 3(1): e001570.

Duckett, S. (1999) 'Policy challenges for the Australian health care system', *Australian Health Review*, 22(2): 130–147.

Duncan, A. E., Ziobrowski, H. N. and Nicol, G. (2017) 'The prevalence of past 12-month and lifetime DSM-IV eating disorders by BMI category in US men and women', *European Eating Disorder Review*, 25(3): 165–171.

Emanuel, L., Berwick, D., Conway, J. et al. (2008) 'What exactly is patient safety?', in K. Henriksen, J. B. Battles and M. A. Keyes (eds) *Advances in Patient Safety: New Directions and Alternative Approaches* (Vol. 1: *Assessment*), Rockville, MD: Agency for Healthcare Research and Quality.

Emparanza, J. I., Cabello, J. B. and Burls, A. J. E. (2015) 'Does evidence-based practice improve patient outcomes? An analysis of a natural experiment in a Spanish hospital', *Journal of Evaluation in Clinical Practice*, 21(6): 1059–1065.

Epstein, R. M. and Street, R. L. (2011) 'The values and value of patient-centered care', *Annals of Family Medicine*, 9(2): 100–103.

Esch, B. M., Marian, F., Busato, A. and Heusser, P. (2008) 'Patient satisfaction with primary care: an observational study comparing anthroposophic and conventional care', *BMC Health Quality of Life Outcomes*, 6: 74.

Fiandt, K. (2006) 'The chronic care model: description and application for practice', *Topics in Advanced Practice Nursing*, 6(4): n.p.

Foley, H. and Steel, A. (2017a) 'Patient perceptions of clinical care in complementary medicine: a systematic review of the consultation experience', *Patient Education and Counselling*, 100(2): 212–223.

Foley, H. and Steel, A. (2017b) 'Patient perceptions of patient-centred care, empathy and empowerment in complementary medicine clinical practice: a cross-sectional study', *Advances in Integrative Medicine*, 4(1): 22–30.

Foley, H. and Steel, A. (2017c) 'The nexus between patient-centered care and complementary medicine: allies in the era of chronic disease?', *Journal of Alternative and Complementary Medicine*, 23(3): 158–163.

Franzel, B., Schwiegershausen M., Heusser, P. and Berger, B. (2013) 'Individualised medicine from the perspectives of patients using complementary therapies: a meta-ethnography approach', *BMC Complementary and Alternative Medicine*, 13(1): 124.

Gollschewski, S., Kitto, S., Anderson, D. and Lyons-Wall, P. (2008) 'Women's perceptions and beliefs about the use of complementary and alternative medicines during menopause', *Complementary Therapies in Medicine*, 16(3): 163–168.

Greene, S. M., Tuzzio, L. and Cherkin, D. (2012) 'A framework for making patient-centered care front and center', *Permanente Journal*, 16(3): 49–53.

Hasnain, M., Connell, K. J., Menon, U. and Tranmer, P. A. (2011) 'Patient-centered care for Muslim women: provider and patient perspectives', *Journal of Women's Health*, 20(1): 73–83.

Hayes, R. D., Dennerstein, L., Bennett, C. M. and Fairley, C. K. (2008) 'What is the "true" prevalence of female sexual dysfunctions and does the way we assess these conditions have an impact?', *Journal of Sexual Medicine*, 5(4): 777–787.

Herman, P.M., Poindexter, B.L., Witt, C.M. and Eisenberg, D.M. (2012) 'Are complementary therapies and integrative care cost-effective? A systematic review of economic evaluations', *BMJ Open*, 2(5): p.e001046.

Hewa, S. and Hetherington, R. W. (1995) 'Specialists without spirit: limitations of the mechanistic biomedical model', *Theoretical Medicine*, 16(2): 129–139.

Hodnett, E. D. (2002) 'Pain and women's satisfaction with the experience of childbirth: a systematic review', *American Journal of Obstetrics and Gynecology*,186(5): S160–S172.

Kautzky-Willer, A. and Harreiter, J. (2017) 'Sex and gender differences in therapy of type 2 diabetes', *Diabetes Research and Clinical Practice*, 131: 230–241.

Kressin, N. R., Skinner, K., Sullivan, L. and Miller, D. R. (1999) 'Patient satisfaction with Department of Veterans Affairs health care: do women differ from men?', *Military Medicine*, 164(4): 283.

Lauby-Secretan, B., Loomis, D. and Straif, K. (2015) 'Breast-cancer screening: viewpoint of the IARC Working Group', *New England Journal of Medicine*, 373(15): 1479.

Leach, M. J. (2010) *Clinical Decision Making in Complementary and Alternative Medicine*, Sydney: Churchill Livingstone.

Leach, M. J. (2013) 'Profile of the complementary and alternative medicine workforce across Australia, New Zealand, Canada, United States and United Kingdom', *Complementary Therapies in Medicine*, 21(4): 364–378.

Leach, M. J. and Gillham, D. (2011) 'Are complementary medicine practitioners implementing evidence based practice?', *Complementary Therapies in Medicine*, 19(3): 128–136.

Leach, M. J. and Tucker, B. (2017a) 'Current understandings of the research-practice gap from the viewpoint of complementary medicine academics: a mixed-method investigation', *Explore*, 13(1): 53–61.

Leach, M. J. and Tucker, B. (2017b) 'Current understandings of the research-practice gap in nursing: a mixed-method study', *Collegian*, In press.

Levesque, J. F., Harris, M. F. and Russell, G. (2013) 'Patient-centred access to health care: conceptualising access at the interface of health systems and populations', *International Journal of Equity in Health*, 12: 18.

Linde, K., Berner, M. M. and Kriston, L. (2008) 'St John's wort for major depression', *Cochrane Database of Systematic Reviews*, (4): CD000448.

Lohr, K. (1990) 'Committee to design a strategy for quality review and assurance', in Medicare (ed.) *Medicare: A Strategy for Quality Assurance*. Vol. 1, Washington, DC: National Academy Press.

Maben, J. (2014) 'Care, compassion and ideals: patient and health care providers' experiences', in S. Shea, R.Wynyard and C. Lionis (eds) *Providing Compassionate Healthcare: Challenges in Policy and Practice*, London: Routledge.

Maciosek, M. V., Coffield, A. B., Flottemesch, T. J., Edwards, N. M. and Solberg, L. I. (2010) 'Greater use of preventive services in US health care could save lives at little or no cost', *Health Affairs*, 29(9): 1656–1660.

Meurk, C., Broom, A., Adams, J. and Sibbritt, D. (2013) 'Bodies of knowledge: Nature, holism and women's plural health practices', *Health*, 17(3): 300–318.

Morgen, S. (2002) *Into Our Own Hands: The Women's Health Movement in the United States, 1969–1990*, New Brunswick, NJ: Rutgers University Press.

Nieuwenhuijze, M. and Low, L. K. (2013) 'Facilitating women's choice in maternity care', *Journal of Clinical Ethics*, 24(3): 276–282.

Nissen, N. (2011) 'Challenging perspectives: women, complementary and alternative medicine, and social change', *Interface*, 3: 187–212.

Olsson, L. E., Jakobsson, E., Swedberg, K. and Ekman, I. (2013) 'Efficacy of person-centred care as an intervention in controlled trials – a systematic review', *Journal of Clinical Nursing*, 22(3–4): 456–465.

Pappa, E., Kontodimopoulos, N., Papadopoulos, A., Tountas, Y. and Niakas, D. (2013) 'Investigating unmet health needs in primary health care services in a representative sample of the Greek population', *International Journal of Environmental Research in Public Health*, 10(5): 2017–2027.

Parrish, R. G. (2010) 'Measuring population health outcomes', *Preventing Chronic Disease*, 7(4): A71.

Pavlish, C. L., Noor, S. and Brandt, J. (2010) 'Somali immigrant women and the American health care system: discordant beliefs, divergent expectations, and silent worries', *Social Science and Medicine*, 71(2): 353–361.

Petroski, E. L., Pelegrini, A. and Glaner, M. F. (2012) 'Reasons and prevalence of body image dissatisfaction in adolescents', *Ciência & Saúde Coletiva*, 17(4): 1071–1077.

Prakash, B. (2010) 'Patient satisfaction', *Journal of Cutaneous and Aesthetetic Surgery*, 3(3): 151–155.

Pressman, S. D., Kraft, T. and Bowlin, S. (2013) 'Well-being: physical, psychological, social', in M. D. Gellman and J. R. Turner (eds) *Encyclopedia of Behavioral Medicine*, New York: Springer.

Puthussery, S. (2016) 'Perinatal outcomes among migrant mothers in the United Kingdom: is it a matter of biology, behaviour, policy, social determinants or access to health care?' *Best Practice & Research Clinical Obstetrics & Gynaecology*, 32: 39–49.

Radwin, L. E. and Alster, K. (2002) 'Individualized nursing care: an empirically generated definition', *International Nursing Review*, 49(1): 54–63.

Rathert, C., Wyrwich, M. D. and Boren, S. A. (2012) 'Patient-centered care and outcomes: a systematic review of the literature', *Medical Care Research and Review*, 70(4): 351–379.

Ried, K., Toben, C. and Fakler, P. (2014) 'Effect of garlic on serum lipids: an updated meta-analysis', *Nutritional Review*, 71(5): 282–299.

Rouse, W. B. (2008) 'Health care as a complex adaptive system: implications for design and management', *Bridge-Washington-National Academy of Engineering*, 38(1): 17.

Saville, A. M. (2015) 'Cervical cancer prevention in Australia: planning for the future', *Cancer Cytopathology*, 124(4): 235–240.

Shaw, D., Guise, J.M., Shah, N. et al. (2016) 'Drivers of maternity care in high-income countries: can health systems support woman-centred care?', *Lancet*, 388(10057): 2282–2295.

Shen, G. C. and Snowden, L. R. (2014) 'Institutionalization of deinstitutionalization: a cross-national analysis of mental health system reform', *International Journal of Mental Health Systems*, 8: 47.

Smith, P. C. (2012) 'What is the scope for health system efficiency gains and how can they be achieved?', *Eurohealth*, 18(3): 3–6.

Steel, A., Adams, J. and Sibbritt, D. (2017) 'The characteristics of women who use complementary medicine while attempting to conceive: results from a nationally representative sample of 13,224 Australian women', *Women's Health Issues*, 27(1): 67–74.

Steel, A., Adams, J., Sibbritt, D. et al. (2012) 'Utilisation of complementary and alternative medicine (CAM) practitioners within maternity care provision: results from a nationally representative cohort study of 1,835 pregnant women', *BMC Pregnancy and Childbirth*, 12(1): 146.

Steel, A., Lucke, J., Reid, R. and Adams, J. (2016) 'A systematic review of women's and health professionals' attitudes and experience of preconception care service delivery', *Family Practice*, 33(6): 588–595.

Stoto, M. A. (2014) 'Population health measurement: applying performance measurement concepts in population health settings', *EGEMS (Washington, DC)*, 2(4): 1132.

Tasca, C., Rapetti, M., Carta, M. G. and Fadda, B. (2012) 'Women and hysteria in the history of mental health', *Clinical Practice and Epidemiology in Mental Health*, 8: 110–119.

Teutsch, S. M., Herman, A. and Teutsch, C. B. (2016) 'How a population health approach improves health and reduces disparities: the case of head start', *Preventing Chronic Disease*, 13: 150565.

Tynkkynen, L. K., Chydenius, M., Saloranta, A. and Keskimäki, I. (2016) 'Expanding choice of primary care in Finland: much debate but little change so far', *Health Policy*, 120(3): 227–234.

Wardle, J., Lui, C. and Adams, J. (2012) 'Complementary and alternative medicine in rural communities: current research and future directions', *Journal of Rural Health*, 28(1): 101–112.

Williams, L. (2015) *The NHS Constitution*, London: Department of Health.

Wilson, D. R. (2010) 'Health consequences of childhood sexual abuse', *Perspectives in Psychiatric Care*, 46(1): 56–64.

Wilson-Stronks, A., Lee, K. K., Cordero, C. L., Kopp, A. L. and Galvez, E. (2008) *One Size Does Not Fit All: Meeting the Health Care Needs of Diverse Populations*, Oakbrook Terrace: The Joint Commission.

Wolf, J. A., Niederhauser, V., Marshburn, D. and LaVela, S. L. (2014) 'Defining patient experience', *Patient Experience Journal*, 1(1): 3.

World Health Organization (2013) *WHO Traditional Medicine Strategy. 2014–2023.* Geneva: World Health Organization.

Worrall, G., Chaulk, P. and Freake, D. (1997). 'The effects of clinical practice guidelines on patient outcomes in primary care: a systematic review', *Canadian Medical Association Journal*, 156(12): 1705–1712.

# Index